Modeling and Simulating Bodies and Garments

Nadia Magnenat-Thalmann

Editor

Modeling and Simulating Bodies and Garments

With contributions by:
Ugo Bonanni, Mustafa Kasap, Bart Kevelham, Mingyu Lim, Christiane Luible, Etienne Lyard, Nadia Magnenat-Thalmann, Dimitris Protopsaltou, Pascal Volino

Visuals by:
Marlène Arévalo-Poizat, Nedjma Cadi-Yazli, Christiane Luible

Springer

Editor
Dr. Nadia Magnenat-Thalmann
Université de Genève
MIRALab
Route de Drize 7
1227 Carouge (Genève)
Switzerland
thalmann@miralab.ch

Cover Image: Marlène Arévalo-Poizat, Nedjma Cadi-Yazli
Editorial Assistance: Ugo Bonanni, Jody Hausmann

ISBN 978-1-4471-5741-0 ISBN 978-1-84996-263-6 (eBook)
DOI 10.1007/978-1-84996-263-6
Springer London Dordrecht Heidelberg New York

British Library Cataloguing in Publication Data
A catalogue record for this book is available from the British Library

Printed on acid-free paper

Springer is part of Springer Science+Business Media (www.springer.com)

Preface

This book contains the research on modeling bodies, cloth and character based adaptation performed during the last 3 years at MIRALab at the University of Geneva. More than ten researchers have worked together in order to reach a truly 3D Virtual Try On. What we mean by Virtual Try On is the possibility of anyone to give dimensions on her predefined body and obtain her own sized shape body, select a 3D cloth and see oneself animated in Real-Time, walking along a catwalk. Some systems exist today but are unable to adapt to body dimensions, have no real-time animation of body and clothes. A truly system on the web of Virtual Try On does not exist so far. This book is an attempt to explain how to build a 3D Virtual Try On system which is now very much in demand in the clothing industry.

To describe this work, the book is divided into five chapters. The first chapter contains a brief historical background of general deformation methods. It ends with a section on the 3D human body scanner systems that are used both for rapid prototyping and statistical analyses of the human body size variations.

Chapter 2 reviews techniques to efficiently and accurately animate virtual humans. The techniques described here enable to tailor the animation to specific subjects, including their shape, and weight characteristics. These animations can then be used to produce virtual catwalks, which in turn can be used as a basis for a Virtual Try On application.

In Chapter 3, methods for measuring the physical parameters of textile materials are described. The core of the chapter is given by the section on the physical simulation of cloth. The addressed topics range from the generalities of mechanical simulation and state-of-the-art techniques to the description of a simple method for accurate simulation of nonlinear cloth materials, covering also numerical integration, collision handling and real-time animation issues. The chapter ends with a section on the haptic interaction with virtual textiles which describes the problems to solve when touching cloth-like deformable objects in a virtual reality environment. It includes a case study detailing the research and development of a prototype interface designed for the haptic simulation of cloth.

The next chapter describes how to design and prototype garments before the manufacturing process. Designers create 3D clothes based on 2D patterns which are either imported from CAD systems or created manually. This process is presented on a case study showing the making of the award winning film "High Fashion in Equations".

The last chapter deals with real life applications as virtual garment prototyping. A discussion addresses current design and manufacturing paradigms and the online customization of garment. A practical example of such online customization is demonstrated by means of MIRALab's Virtual Try On. The chapter finishes with a technical proposal of a virtual garment platform enabling co-design, ranging from low-level communication to higher level user-management.

The book is presented with a lot of images and additional videos can be seen on www.miralab.ch.

Contents

List of Figures

Chapter 1
Modeling Bodies

Abstract This chapter addresses human body modeling techniques and their application fields. After a brief historic background of general deformation methods, they are classified and extended under the following titles: geometric, physically based, anthropometric and anatomic approaches. The chapter ends with a section on the 3D human body scanner systems, that are used both for rapid prototyping and statistical analyses of the human body size variations.

1.1 Introduction

Over the last 3 decades there have been significant hardware and software developments in computer graphics. This progression has mainly focused on achieving realism in virtual environments. Depending on the functionality of each element in virtual environments, efficient shading, skinning, and motion algorithms are developed to simulate their physical properties. Most of these techniques are focused on human body models, which are very important elements of these environments. There are various stages of making virtual bodies, including designing the mesh clone and post stages like shading and skinning. Completing these stages requires a lot of design time but playing these realistic virtual characters in a virtual environment also requires computation power. Due to a bottleneck in the computation power of the PC, it may be necessary to sacrifice the production quality of one or more of the virtual body making stages in order to have an efficient visualization.

One of the most recent techniques for body model generation is to use 3D body scanners to acquire a virtual clone of the original model. This technique can capture data with a resolution of a few millimetres and the final output of the scanner is a single static mesh with a few million vertices. In environments such as the gaming and virtual worlds, it is not possible or efficient to use such massive data since it requires powerful hardware for processing. For the sake of efficiency, it is clearly evident that most of the applications sacrifice realism to achieve the computationally optimal representation of the virtual body by reducing the acquired polygon number.

N. Magnenat-Thalmann (ed.), *Modeling and Simulating Bodies and Garments*,
DOI 10.1007/978-1-84996-263-6_1, © Springer-Verlag London Limited 2010

A cheaper alternative approach for the 3D data acquisition method is to use a set of 2D images taken from different camera views. Special algorithms and heuristics are used to combine these images to generate the 3D resemblance of the model. However, the output quality of this approach is not comparable to the ones generated with 3D body scanners. This method requires professional user interaction and the results are generally not visually satisfactory.

Another way to generate body models is to design them from scratch by means of 3D design tools. When using either data acquisition or designing methods to make the bodies, the resulting production is just a static mesh if the subsequent design stages are not applied. To add further realism, these models are animated by applying walk, grasp etc. motions and then shaders are applied to simulate the skin surface behaviour under different light conditions. The animation of a model is achieved by attaching model specific skinning information on the mesh. Once the skinning process is completed, then it is possible to animate the model with the existing motion capture data. When generating different sizes and types of body models there are two options; body databases are constructed or different variations are created from a single template model.

Body modeling approaches can be classified under two main headings, structural and mathematical (Fig. 1.18). In a structural approach either anthropometry or anatomy knowledge is used to design model variations. In a mathematical approach, physical or geometrical methods are used to parametrically represent the skin surface or underlying layer by polygons, metaballs or soft objects. In most cases, combinations of these methods are used to generate the final model. In the design stage, the body is given a generic shape by using the anthropometric constraints such as the ratio of the body, the height to the limbs or the upper arm length to the lower arm length etc. When the generic model has been designed, anatomical constraints are used to give detailed surface representation like muscle bulging or fatness. As an example, while the belly, breast or muscles are modelled by geometry based methods, a finite element method is applied to the initial shape to simulate the physical behaviour in motion.

In the following, we will describe the basics of body modeling approaches using the related state of the art concepts. As an example a simple anthropometric body modeling technique is demonstrated. Finally, the details of a recent body modeling method, using 3D body scanners are also described.

1.2 Geometric Modeling

Modeling real objects in virtual environments is one of the main research topics in computer graphics. Starting with 2D in the early 1950s, we can now model very complex objects in 3D together with their material properties in many environmental conditions. In the past, CAD/CAM programmes used geometric primitives to model the human body. Due to computation constraints, geometric objects like cylinders and spheres are used to represent the body limbs in simulation applications. The main application area was the ergonomic conformity test, which is a way to visualise the human body inside a vehicle under various conditions. One of the few survey articles that traces the history of the field was presented by Requicha in 1982 (Requicha 1982). Recently it became possible to represent a human body model with parametric curves. This required powerful computation resources for realistic visualisation.

To execute performance sensitive applications with commodity computer hardware, it is necessary to balance the thresholds between all the techniques to be used in the final application. For instance, modeling animated virtual bodies together with physically accurate garments requires the integration of appropriate modeling techniques. Since the body shape details are hidden under garments but the rough body contours affect the garment's physical behaviour, using a geometric model of the body with physical garment modeling techniques gives an optimal performance.

1.2.1 Basic Geometric Deformations

One of the earliest works that may be considered as a milestone in the geometric modeling field is represented by Barr (Barr 1984). During that period, simple geometric primitives were used in model design applications to construct the desired models. Barr introduced super-quadric primitives and angle preserving transformations over the exiting modeling techniques, making it possible to design complex models.

Given two dimensional two curves,

$$s(\omega) = \begin{bmatrix} s_1(\omega) \\ s_2(\omega) \end{bmatrix}, \omega_0 \leqslant \omega \leqslant \omega_1 \quad \text{and} \quad t(\eta) = \begin{bmatrix} t_1(\eta) \\ t_2(\eta) \end{bmatrix}, \eta_0 \leqslant \eta \leqslant \eta_1$$

Barr defines a surface $x(\eta, \omega)$ by a Spherical Cartesian product of these two curves,

$$x(\eta, \omega) = \begin{bmatrix} t_1(\eta) & s_1(\omega) \\ t_1(\eta) & s2(\omega) \\ t_2(\eta) & \end{bmatrix}$$

where ω, η are latitude and longitude parameters of the surface. Using a few sinus, cosines and exponential functions, he modelled super-quadric primitives that are used to construct complex solids. Aside from defining these primitives, he also implemented invertible angle preserving transformations to bend and twist them in three dimensions. These transformation methods simplify the calculation of the new tangent and normal vectors of the surface. In Fig. 1.1 we demonstrate a sample Cartesian product operation to generate a 3D model. A 2D star shape changes its size in the z coordinate to generate the final model.

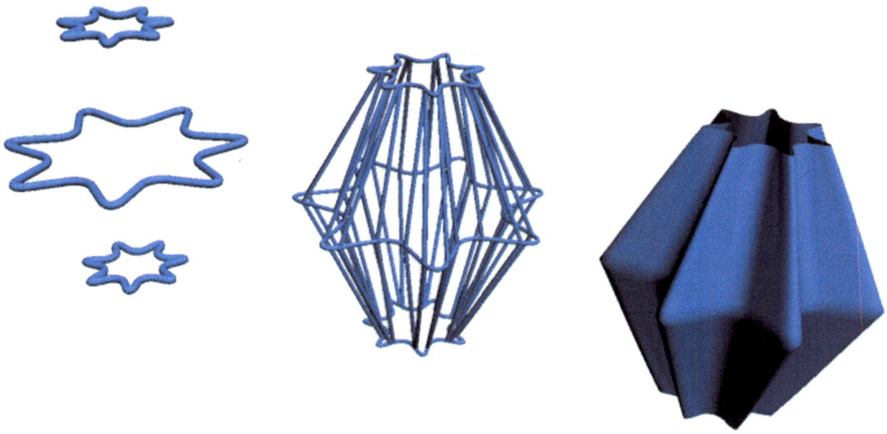

Fig. 1.1 Design of super-quadric primitive by spherical cartesian product

After his successive work on super-quadrics, Barr (1984) developed hierarchical solid modeling operations that simulate twisting, bending and tapering like transformations on geometric objects. The definition of these transformation operations mainly focused on the underlying objects' tangent and normal vector space deformations. Barr provides the general description of the deformation with the following method: If the Jacobean matrix of the deformation function is known, then use it to find the tangent vectors of the original model. Next, apply a tangent transformation on these vectors to find the tangent vectors of the deformed model. Finally, find the deformed model's position vectors with the resulting tangent vectors. Later Barr's definitions inspired researchers to animate human body models by bending the arms and legs and fattening or slimming a specific part of the body by deformation.

Barr's transformation functions are used to achieve axial deformations where only one coordinate of the shape's vertices is operated by the function. Blanc (1994) generalises these functions to achieve global deformations, where each vertex of the model in (the) Euclidian space is mapped to another vertex in the same space. Implemented deformation functions are; pinch, taper, mould, twist, shear and bend. The results of these deformation techniques are represented in Fig. 1.2.

1.2.2 *Free Form Deformation*

Based on Barr's work, Sederberg and Parry (1986) proposed the Free Form Deformation (FFD) technique which is commonly used and has many extensions to solve specific problems related to deformation. In this technique, a grid of arranged point set is embedded on a set of complex objects that will be deformed. Instead of displacing the surface vertices of the objects, a few sets of control points over the grid are displaced. According to the deformation generated on the grid

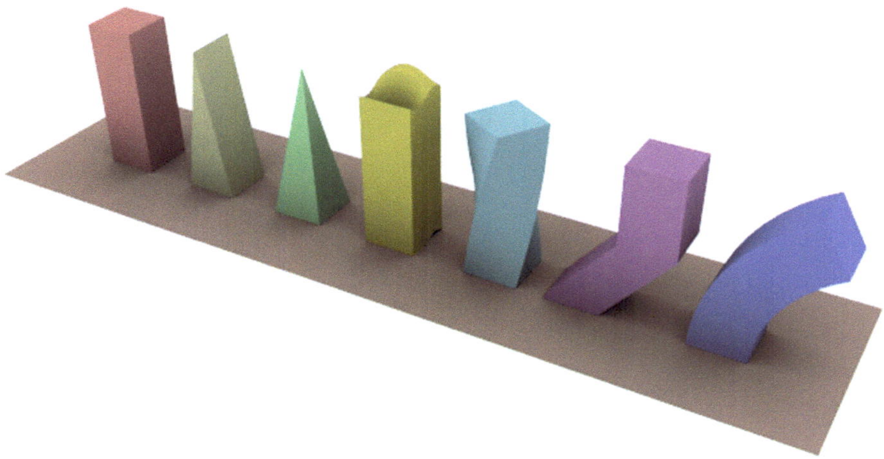

Fig. 1.2 Visual results of global deformations on the leftmost object

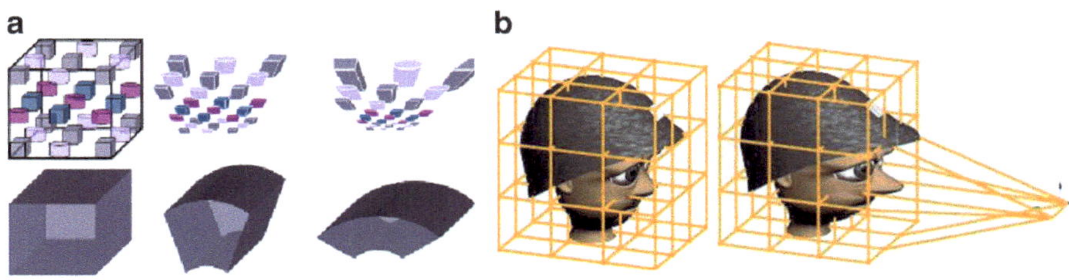

Fig. 1.3 (**a**) FFD based deformation, bending a cube. (**b**) Underlying objects

structure, underlying objects will follow similar deformation behaviour. These procedures are best represented within Fig. 1.3.

In the first row of Fig. 1.3a, a set of original geometric models enclosed within a cube and the deformation of these models along with the enclosed cube can be observed. In the second row only the enclosing cube and the transformation over it are illustrated. More generally in Fig. 1.3b, we can see that displacing the vertices near the nose deforms the character's head.

To make the deformation more flexible, Lamousin (1994) logically extends the FFD by mapping it on a non-uniform rational B-Splines (NURBS) complex instead of a regular grid. NFFD offers much more control over the model, while this was not achieved in the prior FFD implementations. Lamousin demonstrates an interesting application of NFFD with a human leg model as an input (Fig. 1.4).

Forsey (Forsey and Bartels 1988) implemented a refinement approach for manipulating the surface of the models. The refinement process makes it possible to have more control over the surface deformation since it increases the number of control points of the B-Spline surface. Based on this approach, two surface deformation techniques are introduced. The first is a direct modification of the

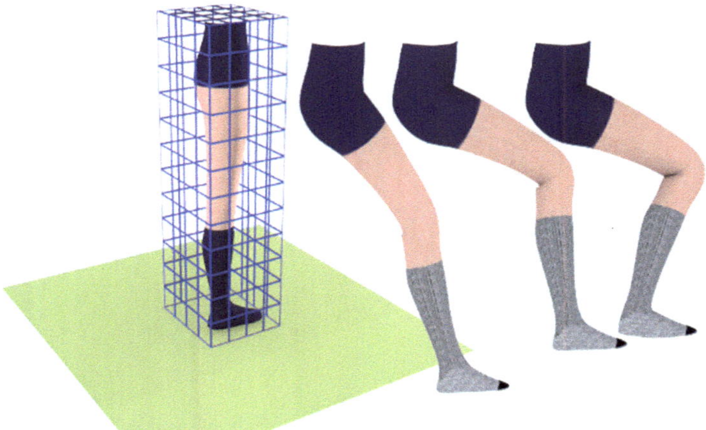

Fig. 1.4 A realistic animation of a human leg with NFFD

control vertices of the surface; the other is called "offset referencing" where the overlaying control vertices are used for refinement.

Forsey used the following terminology for the refinement process:

$$S(u,v) = \sum_i \sum_j V_{i,j} B_{i,k}(u) B_{j,l}(v)$$

Here $S(u,v)$ represents the surface to be modified, $V_{i,j}$ are the control vertices, $B_{i,k}(u), B_{j,l}(v)$ are the basis functions of order k and l. To have more control over this surface, Forsey re-defined the basic functions in a piecewise manner as:

$$B_{i,k}(u) = \sum_r \alpha_{i,k}(r) N_{r,k}(u)$$
$$B_{j,l}(u) = \sum_s \alpha_{j,l}(s) N_{s,l}(v).$$

The original surface is re-defined with more control points by the following formula:

$$S(u,v) = \sum_r \sum_s W_{r,s} N_{r,k}(u) N_{s,l}(v),$$

where

$$W_{r,s} = \sum_i \sum_s \alpha_{i,k}(r) \alpha_{j,l}(s) V_{i,j}.$$

Here $V_{i,j}$ are the control vertices that independently influence a large surface segment for deformation. After a redefinition of the surface, $W_{r,s}$ become the new control points which are more numerous than the original ones.

Figure 1.5a represents the cross section of a surface with the control points in the corresponding section. Figure 1.5b has more control points because of the

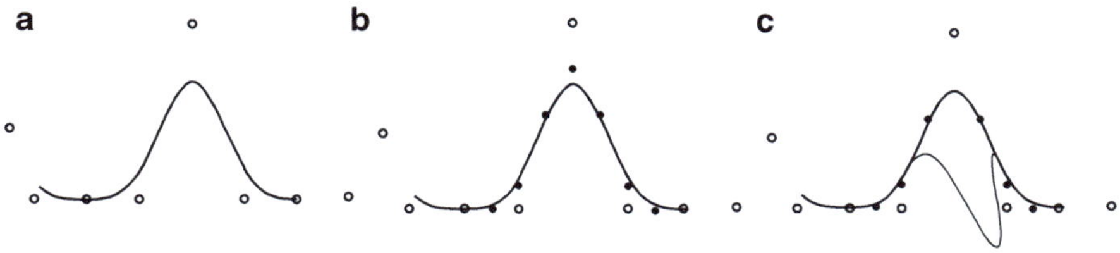

Fig. 1.5 (**a**) A cross section of the original surface with control points. (**b**) Refined version of A. (**c**) Modified surface (Courtesy of David R. Forsey)

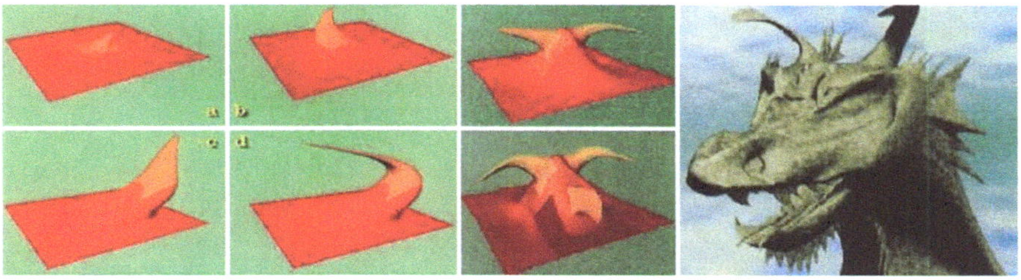

Fig. 1.6 The complex surface is created by the refinement method (Courtesy of David R. Forsey)

refinement. Figure 1.5c represents the deformed version of the surface which cannot be achieved with a low number of control points (Fig. 1.6).

Another interactive deformation technique which has a complete theoretical presentation with mathematical proofs is presented by Borrel (Borrel and Rappoport 1994). In this approach the deformation is considered with two-step calculations. Firstly, the product of polynomial function f in $\Re^n$ into $\Re^m$ is constructed by transforming from the lower space to a higher one ($m > n$). Secondly, a different linear projection is applied to succeed the deformation back from $\Re^m$ into $\Re^n$. During this projection, transformation matrix M is used to generate appropriate deformations.

Figure 1.7 presents the geometric interpretation of a deformation from two to three dimensions and backward. In the figure, the initial two dimensional curve is first transformed into third dimension as a 3D object. Then, transformation matrix M is used to project the 3D object back into 2D with its deformed versions.

Based on FFD, Decaudin (1996) introduced a more interactive technique for modeling shapes from a simple geometric primitive like an ellipse. In this technique a deformation tool composed of a convex shape is located in the space. By using this tool it is possible to produce bump or dent effects on any primitive. This tool can be visualised as a balloon which is inflating inside or outside of the model to give a bump effect (Fig. 1.8). The main disadvantage of this is the amount of user interaction required for the modeling.

Most of these deformation techniques have an unconstrained effect on the applied surface. A new synthesis over the existing FFD techniques is to use Borrel's (Borrel and Rappoport 1994) constrained deformation method. The controlled spatial deformation feature of this method is the main difference. To achieve a desired local deformation, constrained region(s) along with a B-Spline curve(s) are defined.

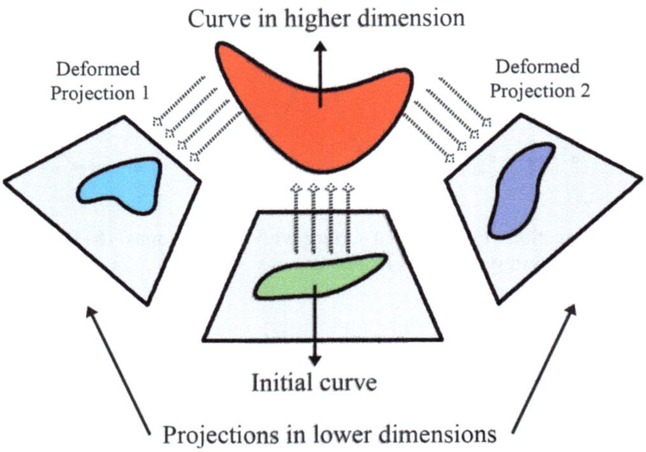

Fig. 1.7 Transformation from lower dimension to upper one and then back to lower one with deformation

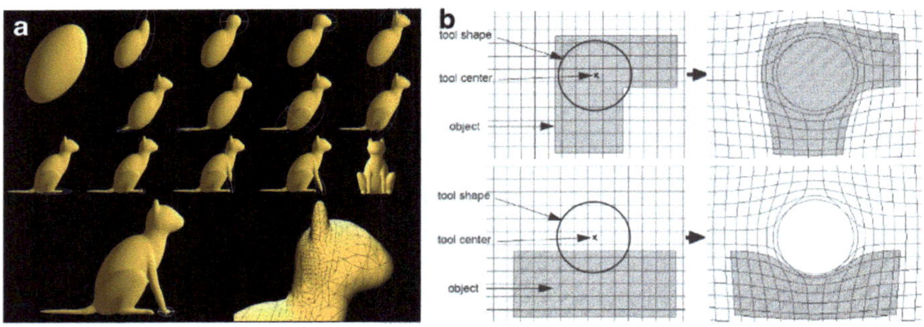

Fig. 1.8 (**a**) From ellipse to cat. (**b**) Deformation tool inside and outside the model (Courtesy of Philippe Decaudin)

In Fig. 1.9, C1 is the centre of the constraint and the circle is the constrained region. $F1$ is an arbitrary deformation function where both ends of the function evolve to zero. The deformation function is defined in [–1, 1] domain and Max(F1(Q)) = 1. Borrel defines the constrained deformation with the following formula:

$$d(Q) = \sum_{i=1}^{r} M_i f_i(Q)$$

r: Number of constraints
Q: Vertex, column order vector
$d(Q)$: Displacement of Q
M_i: Scale column order vector
f_1: Contribution of ith constraint

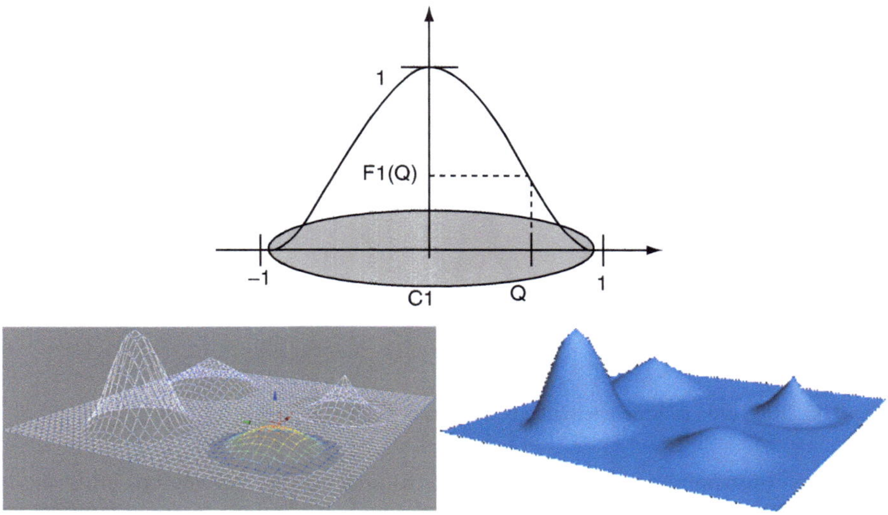

Fig. 1.9 Deformation around the constraint and the resulting effect on a grid

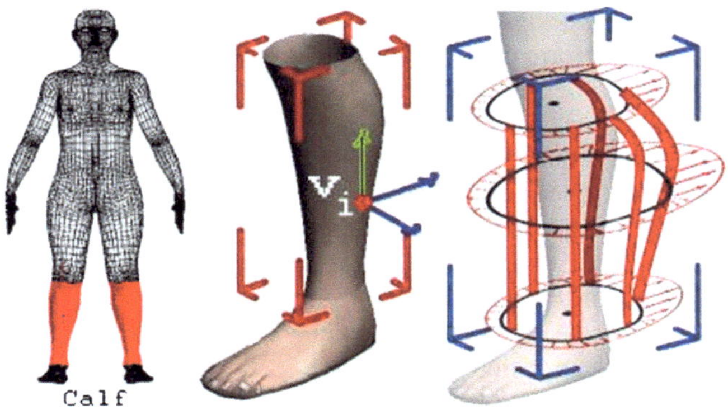

Fig. 1.10 Deforming constrained regions on the body model

By using this approach, one can define small regions with more control and smoothly displace the vertices under the region. During the displacement operation, it is possible to use different types of functions like B-splines to generate a complex deformation within a region.

Figure 1.10 represents the application of a similar method on a specific part of the body region, for instance, the calf. Kasap (Kasap and Magnenat-Thalmann 2007) applied a constrained deformation approach by defining constrained regions to generate different sized body models.

The main difference between this approach and the original one is the dimensions of the region. Instead of defining a constraint in 2D, here volume regions are used. In Fig. 1.10, one of the anthropometric body regions called "calf" is demonstrated

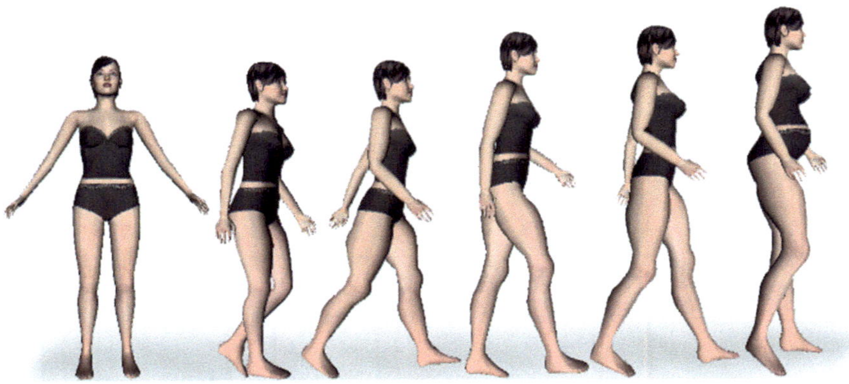

Fig. 1.11 Real-time anthropometric body deformation

with the corresponding constraint volume. Similar to the calf region, other main regions like the arm, belly, thigh etc. are defined. According to some constraints based on Borel's approach, body parts are deformed to generate size range models in real-time as is shown in Fig. 1.11.

Depending on the body region, several B-spline curves are used as a deformation function to achieve the desired body size.

Another type of deformation technique where the result looks similar to the constrained deformation is called "the wires". Singh (Singh and Fiume 1998) inspired by sculptors, used wire curves to give a main deformation schema to a model like armature. Along with the domain curves, wires are used to manipulate an implicit volume. The main advantage of the wire deformation is that it is independent of the complexity of the underlying object. Once it is defined for the base object, then it is appropriate to use it multiple times with varying objects. An application domain example of this technique is represented by modeling a human head. The inverse kinematics technique is used to simulate highly flexible skeletons for wrinkle generation over the face.

The following tuple is used to define a wire deformation: $\langle W, R, s, r, f \rangle$ where

W, R: Free form parametric curves. W wire curve, R reference curve
r: Offset surface distant from a curve
s: Scale factor
f: Density function to calculate the object vertices within an offset volume

Once the wire deformation schema is defined with the above definition, it is possible to make global or local deformations on the model by changing the curve parameters. This is best presented in Fig. 1.12 with local deformations on the face and global deformations on the arm.

Another approach for deformation is applying the sweep based method on a model (Hyun et al. 2003). In this approach, a limb for example is approximated by a sweep based ellipsoid which changes its size as it moves through the limb. Also, the ellipsoid changes its orientation through the joint locations. During this sweep

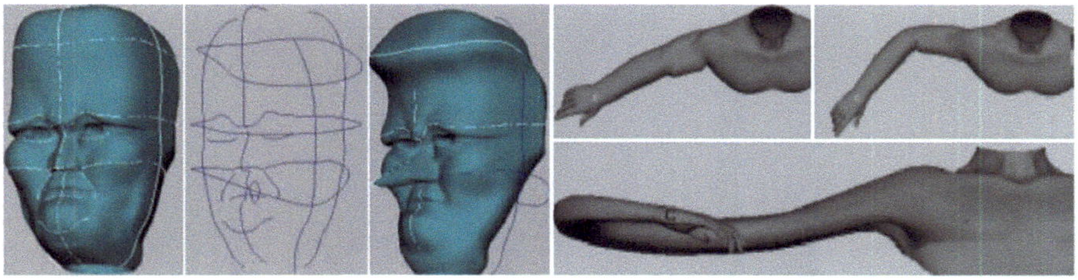

Fig. 1.12 Wires deformation application for head model and inverse kinematics (Courtesy of Karan Singh and Eugene Fiume, Autodesk Inc)

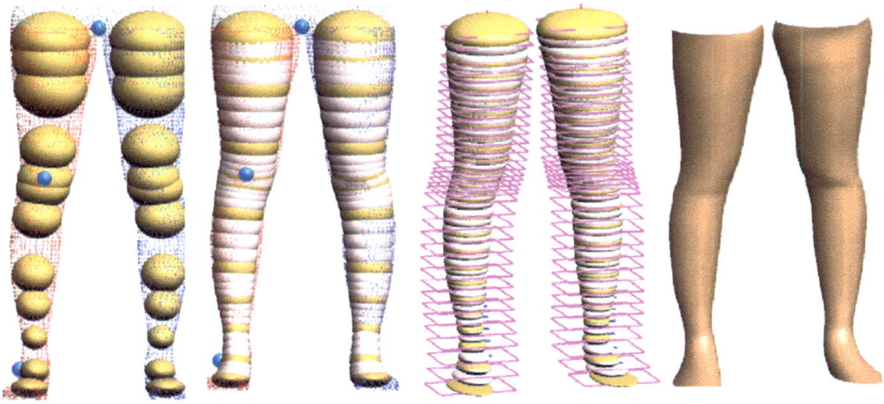

Fig. 1.13 Sweep surface generated by moving ellipsoids (Hyun et al. 2003)

motion, all modified ellipsoids are interpolated to fit in the original model. The resulting approximated model is processed with a displacement map to reflect the original shape because of its smooth behaviour. The stages in this process are presented in Fig. 1.13.

Hyun (Hyun et al. 2003) extended his sweep based approach for body deformation by adding GPU assisted collision detection for limbs during the deformation. A user specified polygonal mesh is first approximated with control sweep surfaces. Second, these sweep surfaces are deformed according to the joint angle changes and finally the overlapping regions are blended. Some anatomical features like elbow-protrusion, skin folding, etc. are emulated in the GPU.

A recent geometric muscle deformation technique was presented by Pratscher in 2005 (Pratscher et al. 2005). The main idea was to use multi-shell structured ellipsoids to produce visually realistic models, as in Fig. 1.14. Each shell has its own level of hardness in order to deform the attached skin. Using a number of heuristics, body mesh is partitioned into segments to determine the location of the muscles. The developed system is capable of customising the muscle connections, size etc. and those parameters saved under a musculoskeletal template, then, can be applied on different bodies. Muscle mapping on the body with a single pose or multiple poses is also considered.

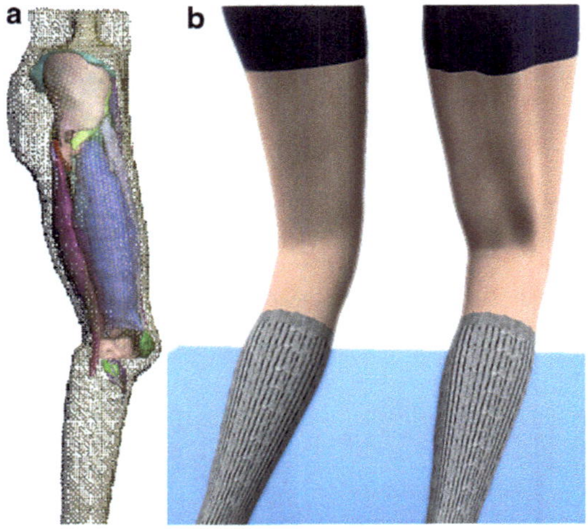

Fig. 1.14 (**a**) Template musculature mapped on the leg model. (**b**) Skin with/without deformation

1.3 Physically Based Modeling

Increasing the precision of the simulation results in more realistic models. But simulating the details of the skin surface, the dynamic muscle bulging or the fat tissue's behaviour is computationally very complex or not realistic with geometric modeling techniques. Whenever such details are important in a body model generation, the inevitable choice is to use the physical based techniques. However, one must decide about the performance requirements before switching between physical or geometric modeling techniques since physical methods require much more computation power.

The flesh layer of the model mainly requires special modeling techniques to simulate realistic behaviour. Animated models represent the most noticeable flesh deformation since they consist of complicated muscle and fat tissue. Under different conditions like bending the arms, running with a big belly or activities that make the muscles bulge, simulation becomes impossible with the geometric methods. One of the earlier researches about the simulation of physical behaviour in computer graphics is implemented by Terzopoulos (Terzopoulos et al. 1987). They modelled materials such as rubber and cloth with the use of an elasticity theory. Later, this method was used in body modeling with different approaches. Some researchers (Teran et al. 2005) implemented the muscle layer with physics based methods and updated the skin surface mesh according to the deformations generated by the underlying layers. Yet, integrating both geometric and physical methods produces a simulation with optimal performance.

As an example, a physics based body modeling approach is to divide the model into three anthropometric layers: skeleton, muscle and skin. The main objective is to implement an articulated skeleton, physical muscle deformation and a parametric surface for the skin. As an example of this approach, Nedel (Nedel et al. 1998) used the physical deformation process to model the anatomic muscle layer. To represent the efficiency of the implementation, one of the most complex muscles is modelled and deformed by a mass-spring model. Considering two attachment points of the muscles to bones, named origin and insertion, the line between these two endpoints is called the action line. This line is used to mechanically quantify the muscle forces in action. The design of the muscle model is manually generated by using a collection of artistic anatomy pictures and corresponding action lines, as shown in Fig. 1.15. The designed muscle mesh requires a post processing stage to regularise the vertices in the direction of the corresponding action line. Once the muscle model is generated interactively, the skin layer is modelled. Using the ray-casting method, the skin surface is sampled where the sampled points are directly used as a control point of the spline curves. Using this method, each slice is combined to construct the skin surface.

Another approach for physics based muscle modeling is to use tetrahedrons to fill the anatomic body parts. Once this implementation succeeds, the generated model behaves as a flesh body part. Using this method, each tetrahedron can simulate a different physical property to construct a heterogeneous model. As an example, Teran (Teran et al. 2005) segmented the visible human MRI dataset to extract the real muscle shape format. This will be the base envelope for the aforementioned model. Once the muscle shape has been constructed, it is filled with tetrahedrons to apply physical behaviour by means of FEM. Because the tendons and the belly muscle behave differently in their density, different parts of the model are simulated with appropriate tetrahedron material properties. The results of the simulations were much more realistic (Fig. 1.16) than the previously mentioned methods.

The application of physical phenomena to improve the flesh parts of the body is not only constrained to the muscles. Larboulette (Larboulette et al. 2005) proposed a fast and simple technique to enhance the standard character skinning method by adding dynamic skin effects (Fig. 1.17) by using the underlying skeleton. A method called rigid skinning is applied to the existing skinning information without modifying its kinematic deformations or other post processed data. The efficiency of this technique comes from the real-time applicability of the visco-elastic properties of the body parts.

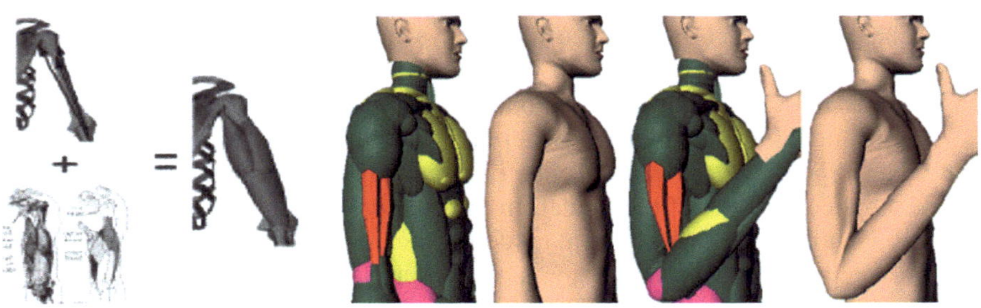

Fig. 1.15 Combination of skeleton and muscle images to construct a 3D model

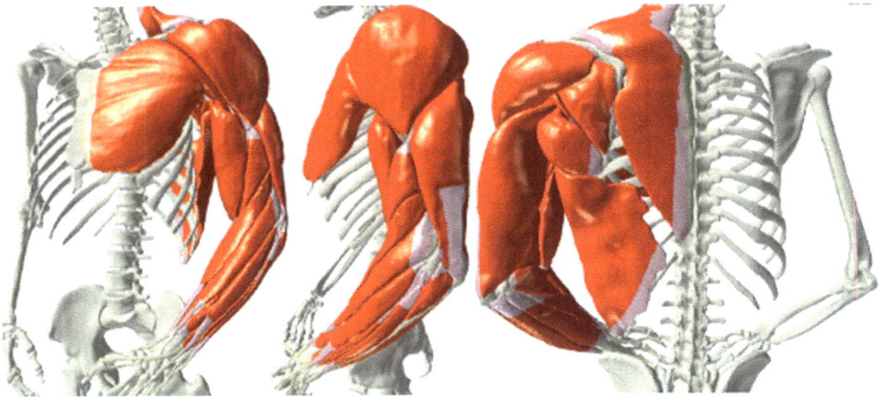

Fig. 1.16 Realistic musculoskeletal model (Courtesy of Joseph M. Teran)

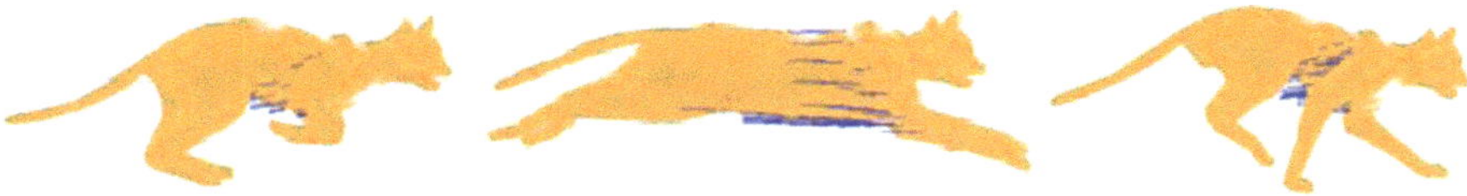

Fig. 1.17 Dynamic skinning effects (Courtesy of Caroline Larboulette)

1.4 Anatomic and Anthropometric Body Modeling Techniques

Early research on human body modeling started in the fifties. In those days, it was important for many organisations that produced aircraft and automobiles etc., due to the need to find the best human body sizes to fit into their products. Later, in the early 1980s, many computer aided design programmes were developed to accelerate this process. Dooley (Dooley 1982) prepared one of the surveys in this field. Later on, with the recent technological developments in the entertainment sector, computer games became one of the main fields to use virtual body models. More recently the textile, medical and sports sectors have been using these virtual models for their products simulation.

In the previous section, geometric and physical modeling techniques are mentioned with their application areas related to the body modeling field. As is represented in Fig. 1.18, high level modeling approaches are considered over these low level modeling techniques. Generally, these anatomic and anthropometric modeling approaches are used together or separately to achieve realism depending on the application area of the model. In the medical research field, realistic body models are simulated with physical modeling techniques. In such applications that require accurate models, an anatomical approach with pure physical modeling produces better results. In case of computational resource constraints, a geometric modeling with anthropometric approach is preferred. Due to the limitations with

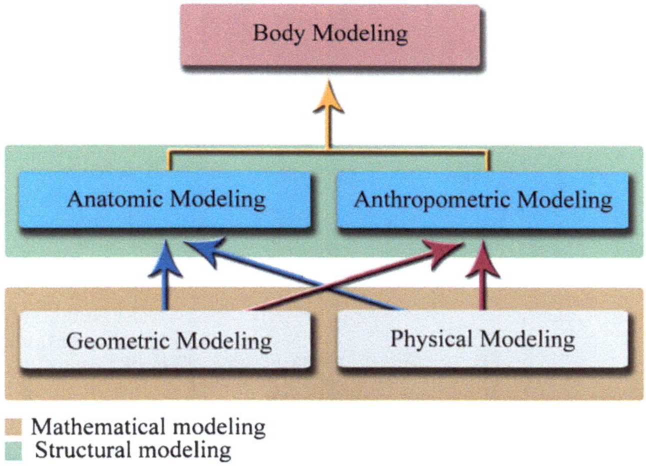

Fig. 1.18 Human body modeling techniques

ordinary computer hardware, it is very important to find the best load balancing parameters in the target application.

Anthropometry is the science of body measurement that focuses on the physical variations of the body size. Considering the importance of human models in virtual environments, anthropometry knowledge is also adapted into computer graphics to parametrically design different size models. These parametric models are used in variety of application fields. For example, textile applications such as virtual Try-on, need anthropometric features to generate a virtual character and to simulate clothes on the character. Also, generating virtual crowds with a variety of realistic characters requires this information for parametric modeling.

Fig. 1.19 represents several anthropometric measurements that are used by designers. Some of these landmarks may differ from one application area to another with different names or order. And some of the measurements can be statistically regenerated from the combination of other measurements. So, these sets of measurements may be decreased to a smaller set or increased to have more variety.

One of the earlier systems that is based on a virtual body model was developed by Magnenat-Thalmann in 1987 (Magnenat-Thalmann and Thalmann 1987). This system was named "the human factory system" and contains both physical and geometrical modeling methods. By means of high level language, synthetic actors are controlled by end users who do not have any programming experience. This system was designed in a modular structure where each module had a specific control or effect on the virtual actor. The complete architecture is shown in Fig. 1.20.

This system contains skeleton control, grasping, and facial animation based on modules which allows a complete body modeling framework. Using this system, authors implemented a scenario of a 7 min film "Rendez-Vous a Montreal" (Magnenat-Thalmann and Thalmann 1987). Nowadays, together with the development of the technology, more complicated visual effects, speech synthesis and

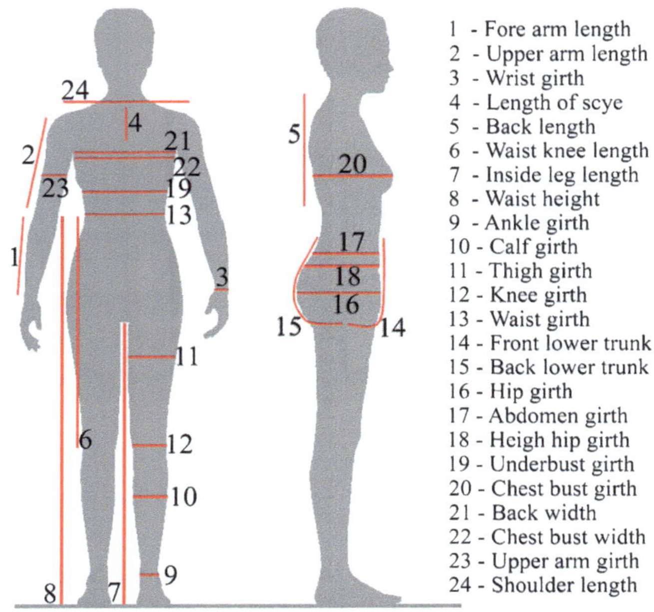

Fig. 1.19 Several anthropometric human body measurements

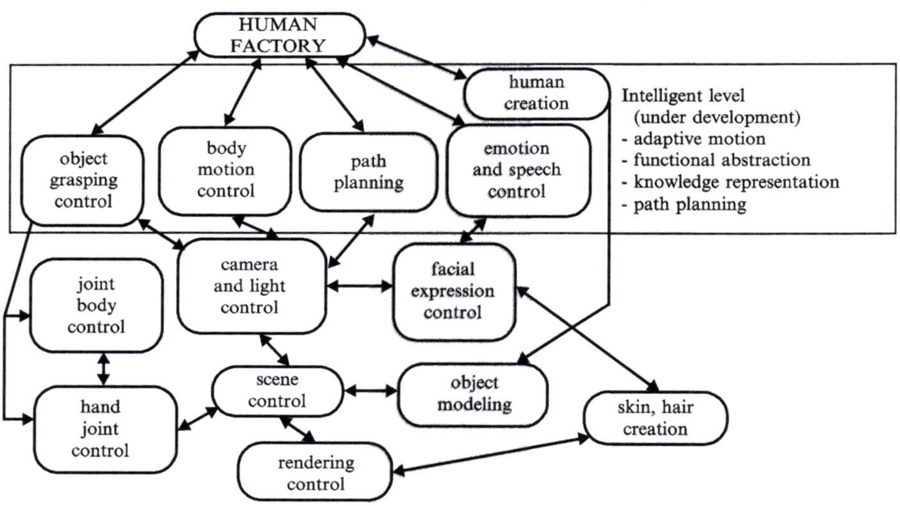

Fig. 1.20 Human factory system architecture

recognition, face detection and recognition like modules are also considered in such systems. Parallel execution of the previously mentioned modules in such systems requires the effective integration of appropriate modeling algorithms.

Deformation of a body model is not only used to generate different size variations. It is also used for animating the body and visualising the physical behaviour over the skin surface etc. Magnenat-Thalmann (Magnenat-Thalmann et al. 1988) developed joint-dependent local deformation (JLD) operators to deform the surface of a model of a human hand for animation. Each JLD operator is affecting its uniquely defined domain and its value is determined as a function of angular values of the joints under a motion. The skeletal structure of the hand is used to implement the joints of the model. Later Magnenat-Thalmann (Magnenat-Thalmann et al. 1988) used the same method for full body animation with the full skeletal joints. The joint hierarchy and the sample implementation are shown in Fig. 1.21.

The basics of the anatomical modeling approach come from Chadwick (Chadwick et al. 1989) who developed a layered model construction method to achieve the visual realism. In this approach, complex body models are designed with parametric constraints that affect the layered structure of the model. For example, a muscle and fatty tissue layer is a mapping from skin data to the underlying skeleton layer. A free form deformation method is used for modeling this layer. A set of prototype deformation operators is provided for skin deformation through muscle abstraction. Each muscle is represented by a pair of FFD cubes with seven planes of control points where the planes are orthogonal to the link axis. In Fig. 1.22, two adjoining FFD cubes are represented where each cube has four planes with one plane shared. Two

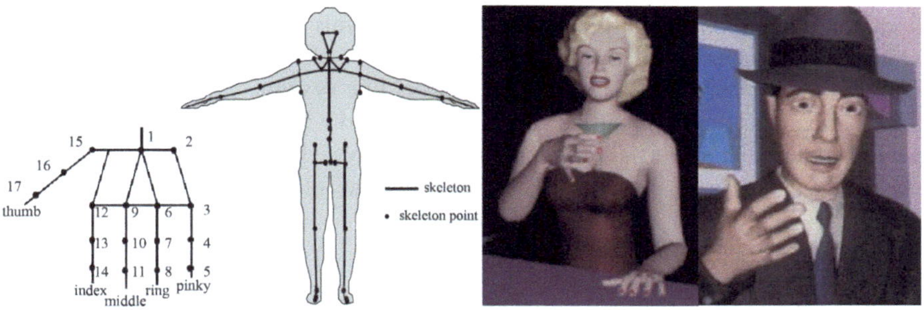

Fig. 1.21 Joints for the hand and the full body and the sample implementation of JLD operators in action

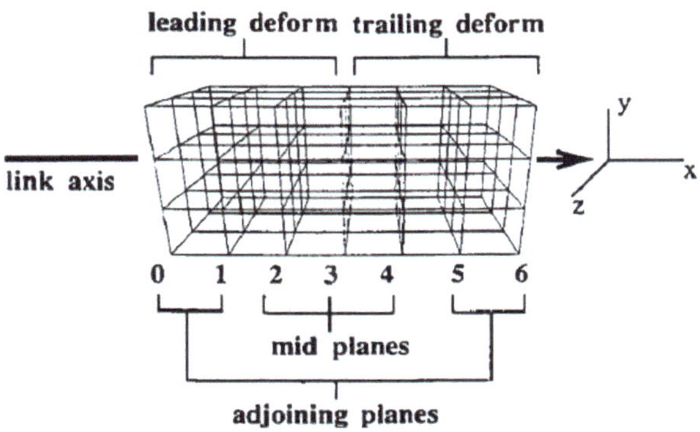

Fig. 1.22 Muscle abstraction through FFD (Courtesy of Richard Parent)

planes at either end provide the continuity between the muscles. Three planes in the middle are used to represent the kinematic and dynamic behaviour of the muscle.

Overall deformations are based on dynamic and kinematic constraints. Kinematic constraints are the skeletal state of the underlying joints that provide the squash and stretch behaviour. The kinesiology literature (Steindler 1955) uses elasticity and contractility properties to define muscle and joint action characteristics. According to these properties, Chadwick developed a set of algorithms to model the flexor and extensor tendon deformation for each frame. After skeletal motion computation, dynamic deformation is applied on the final skin mesh by using a mass-spring approach on the pre-computed FFD cube. The behaviour of the skin surface is shown in Fig. 1.23.

One of the earliest pieces of research about the anthropometric modeling of the human body model was introduced by Azuola in 1994 (Azuola et al. 1994). First, the human body model is segmented into groups according to the synovial joints. Deformation on the corresponding joint is constrained with its degree of freedom (DOF). According to the anthropometric measurement database, the anthropometrically segmented body model is deformed with FFD methods. Azuola developed a system called JAKE that performs shape estimation segmentation and joint determination. The output of the system is used to generate a virtual body constructed with deformable segments. Each segment is a geometric primitive connected by joints which have less than 4 degrees of freedom. Polyhedral human body model segments are uniformly and non-uniformly scaled to construct different sized body models based on the SASS (Azuola et al. 1993) system which is an anthropometric body measurement spreadsheet like system.

Azuola's deformation method can be summarised with the following definitions. Model cantered non-inertial reference frame ϕ is based on inertial reference frame Φ to express a vertex position on the model by the following equation:

$$x = c + R\,p$$

Here $c(t)$ is the centre of the φ, and R(t) is the rotation with respect to Φ. Also local displacement d and global vertex position s are summed to find the final vertex

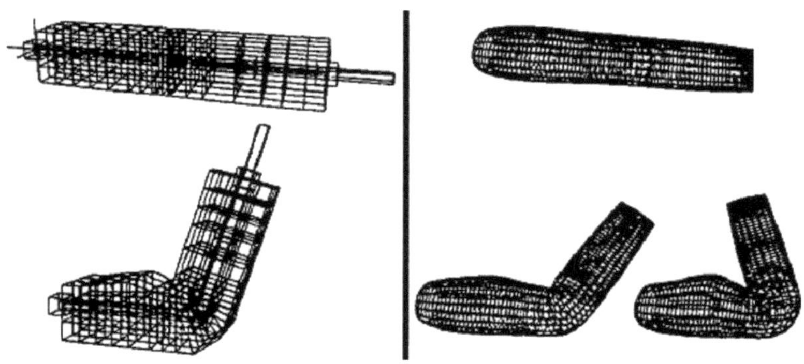

Fig. 1.23 Dynamic muscle effect based on FFD (Courtesy of Richard Parent)

position by $p = s + d$. Under these circumstances, two different postures of two models m_0 and m_1 at time values t and $t + \delta t$ are observed. To find the joint position of the model by using two different postures, Azuola solved the following equations:

$$x_0(t) = c_0(t) + R_0(t)p_0$$
$$x_0(t+\delta t) = c_0(t+\delta t) + R_0(t+\delta t)p_0 \quad \text{for model } m_0$$

and

$$x_1(t) = c_1(t) + R_1(t)p_1$$
$$x_1(t+\delta t) = c_1(t+\delta t) + R_1(t+\delta t)p_1 \quad \text{for model } m_1$$

It is assumed that these models m_0 and m_1 are in the same posture at the same time intervals. With this precondition, the equation becomes:

$$x_0(t) = x_1$$
$$x_0(t+\delta t) = x_1(t+\delta t)$$

and

$$\begin{bmatrix} R_0(t) & -R_1(t) \\ R_0(t+\delta t) & -R_1(t+\delta t) \end{bmatrix} \begin{bmatrix} p_0 \\ p_1 \end{bmatrix} = \begin{bmatrix} c_1(t) - c_0(t) \\ c_1(t+\delta t) - c_0(t+\delta t) \end{bmatrix}$$

Once the joint points have been determined, appropriate FFD deformation can be applied on the body segment, as is presented in Fig. 1.24.

In most cases, polygonal model representation techniques are used but the slice based model construction is also important in deformation methods. Instead of using a polygonal representation, Shen (Shen et al. 1994) divided the model into slices to achieve better deformation results. Each slice is defined with parametric curves, namely B-splines. Depending on the distance of the neighbouring joints and the normal vectors of the slices, collision is prevented. The radius of each contour is scaled to achieve the muscular deformation effect.

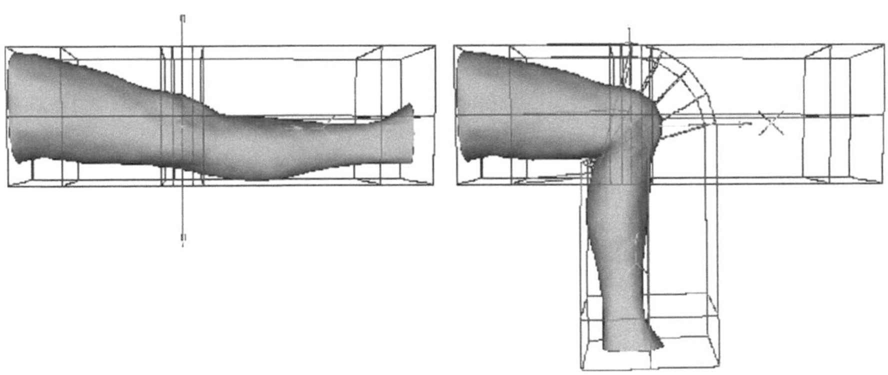

Fig. 1.24 FFD application on body segment (Courtesy of Norman I. Badler)

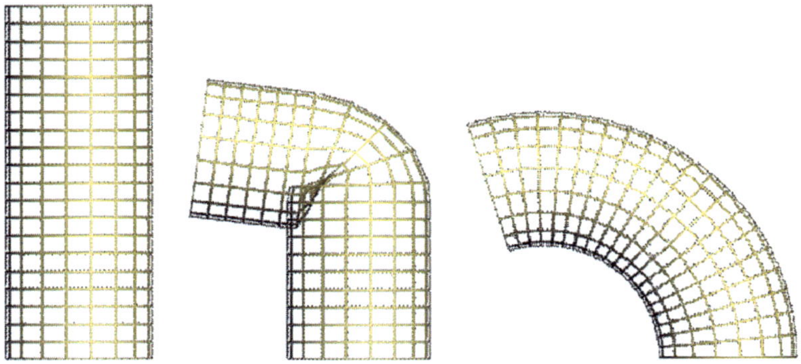

Fig. 1.25 Slice collisions around the joint region

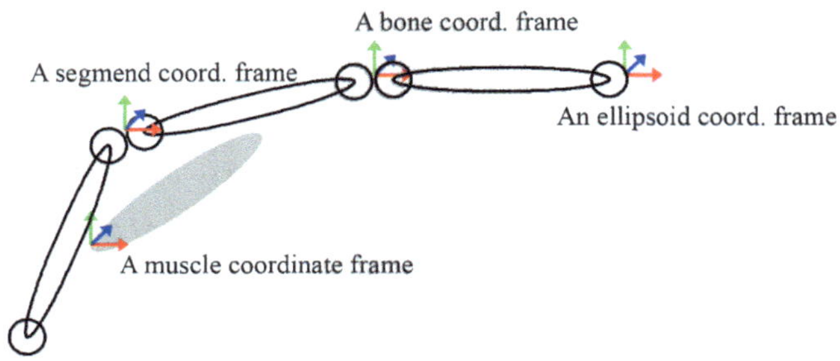

Fig. 1.26 Sample model hierarchy and coordinate frames of nodes

To prevent the slice collision problem, the application of the previously mentioned method is visually summarised using the cylinder model in Fig. 1.25. Using this approach, the body model is divided into the main limbs like the arms, legs and torso. Each limb is deformed like the previously mentioned cylinder model to achieve visually realistic results.

Wilhelms (1995) implemented a new method where the body layers can be defined in a hierarchic structure. This approach makes it possible to add and remove bones, muscles and skin in the hierarchy. The flexibility of this method is used to define several body structures that have a different skeleton and muscle hierarchy. In this multilayered approach, each structure has its own coordinate frame to simplify the computations. Also, ellipsoid models are used instead of the muscle structures for efficiency. A sample structure is represented in Fig. 1.26. According to the interaction of these structures, skin surface is deformed for visually realistic models.

Each muscle between two neighbouring skeletons is modelled with three ellipsoids to construct a real muscle model with two tendons and one muscle belly.

After the muscle hierarchy construction, the initial skin is generated. Using the iterative Newton-Raphson approach, for each skin vertex, the nearest point on

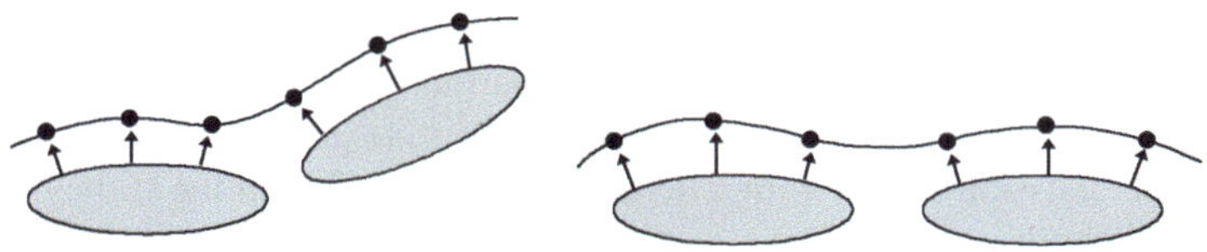

Fig. 1.27 Anchored skin to muscle with rest and extend postures

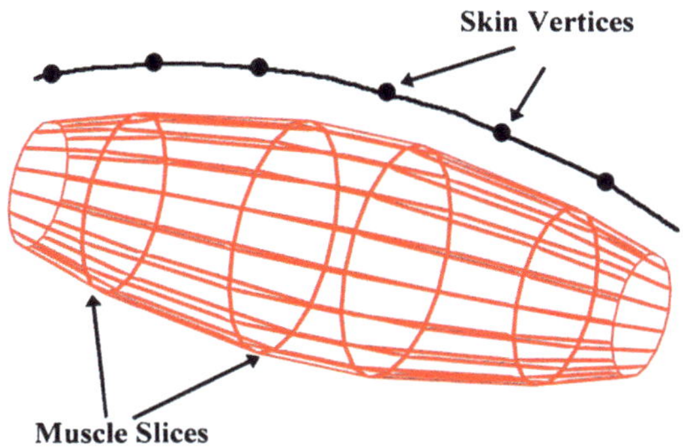

Fig. 1.28 Parametric deformed cylinder for muscle modeling

the ellipse is found. Using this information, skin is anchored to the muscle. According to the motion of the muscles, the skin surface is updated to produce realistic muscle effects on the body. This method is implemented on a cat model where the resulting effects are shown in Fig. 1.27.

The deformed cylinder muscle method, which provides a better compromise between speed and visual realism, is used to model the underlying layers of a skin. The deformed cylinder method is implemented by defining two origins and two insertion locations on a specific bone. These locations are parameterised according to the bounding box of the corresponding bone. This parameterisation makes it possible to use the same implementation on other individuals. Each deformed cylinder is divided by eight elliptic slices to generate muscle segments. These slices are discretised into equally spaced radial points to generate a polygon. Later, neighbouring points on each slice are connected to generate the muscle mesh, as is represented in Fig. 1.28.

Once the insertion and the origin locations of the default muscle are determined by the user, a corresponding deformed cylinder is automatically constructed for further deformations. Non-default muscles such as the ones on the upper arm that are connected to the torso are modelled in a slightly different manner where more user interaction is required. During the animation, the approximate muscle volume preservation is considered. Even if biological volume preservation is not satisfied, current and relaxed volume ratios and muscle lengths are used to recalculate the deformation. Main contribution of this method is the skin deformation with a response to the underlying layers. Since the skin is a triangle mesh surface, it is displaced according to the underlying deformation. The skin's triangle mesh surface is generated by the voxelisation method. Discrete grid points on the body are filtered by a Gaussian kernel with a density function to determine if they are inside or outside the body. According to the user defined threshold, eliminated grid points are used to construct the triangular mesh. The next step is to anchor the skin vertex to the nearest underlying component. This is achieved by associating each skin vertex to the nearest previously created muscle segment. Finally, a series of relaxation operators based on the area of each skin surface polygon are used to achieve the simulation of elastic membrane.

Scheepers (Scheepers et al. 1997) offered an anatomical deformation approach for plausible visual effects where their research is focused on skeletal muscle modeling. Structurally skeletal muscles consist of three parts; namely the belly, origin and insertion part. For the belly part of the skeletal muscle, they used ellipsoidal modeling with the following formulas, where a, b and c represent the parameters of the ellipse in three axes:

$l = 2c$: is the length of the muscle.

$r = \frac{a}{b}$: is the ration of height to width.

$v = \frac{4\pi abc}{3} = \frac{4\pi rb^2 c}{3}$: is the volume of the ellipse.

$l' = 2c'$: is the new length of the muscle after deformation.

$b' = \sqrt{\frac{3v}{4\pi rc'}}, a' = b'r$: are the new width and height of the muscle belly.

Using the above formulation, $r = (1 - t)r_n + ktr_n = (1 - t + kt)r_n$ gives the new height/width ratio of the muscle belly where r_n is the ratio in a relaxed state. Here t is the tension ratio parameter and k is the tension control parameter. Scheepers offered to set $k = 2.56$for visually realistic modeling. Figure 1.29 represents the state of the muscle with parameter $t = 0$ and $t = 1$.

Two types of skeletal muscle model are considered, the first is the widely used simple form called fusiform that behaves like straight lines and the second, which is more complex is multi-belly muscles, which is modelled as tubular shaped

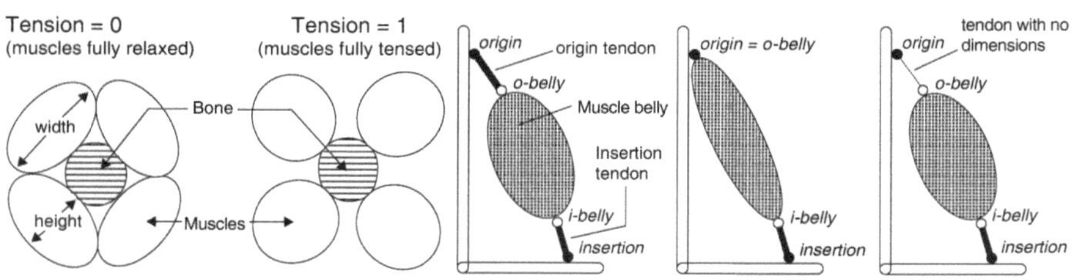

Fig. 1.29 Muscle deformation (Courtesy of Richard Parent)

bi-cubic patch meshes capped with elliptic hemispheres. Based on these modeling primitives, Scheepers developed a procedural language to describe an anatomical model. A sample implementation on the arms and torso is shown in Fig. 1.30.

Another example for anthropometry based deformation comes from DeCarlo et al. (1998) Their system automatically generates new face models from a collection of anthropometric measurements and their statistical analyses. These anatomical measurements are mainly used as constraints on a parameterised template surface. To achieve the constrained surface generation, variational modeling techniques are used. The term, measure of fairness is used to detect the quality of the modeling where it formalises how much the surface resembles the desired one. Anthropometric measurements for deformation are generated by first identifying the particular landmarks on the model surface. A series of measurements between these landmarks generate the anthropometric measurement collection. A dependency graph of the measurements is constructed to find which measurement parameter is affected by the other one. The results are used to deform the B-Spline surface which is the optimal shape representation for the variational and anthropometrical modeling technique. Figure1.31 represents the landmarks used to generate an anthropometric measurement collection and randomly generated face models.

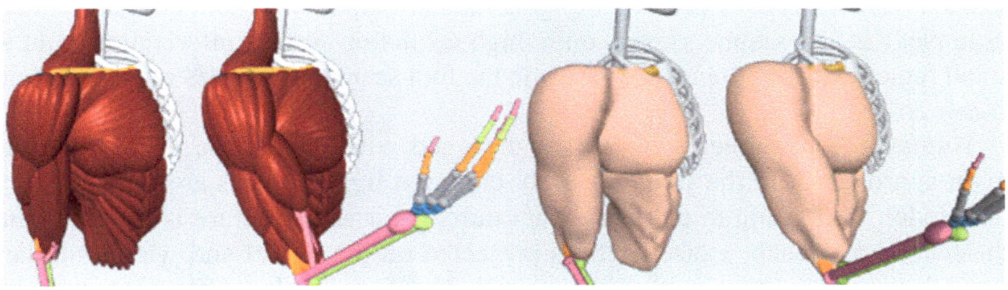

Fig. 1.30 Muscle modeling on upper arm (Courtesy of Richard Parent)

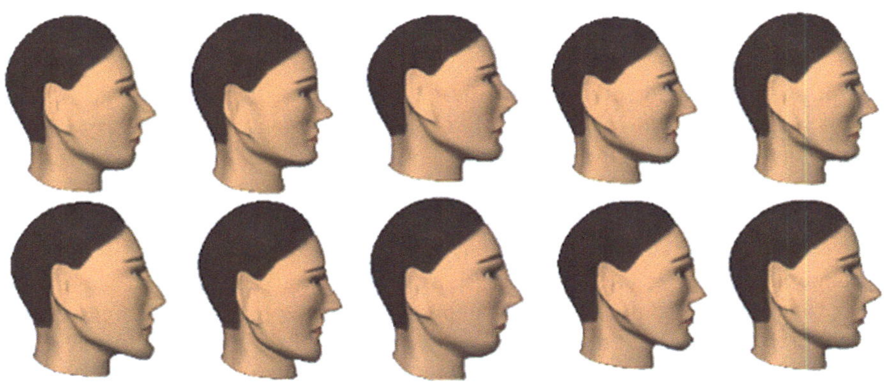

Fig. 1.31 Variational and anthropometric modeling (Courtesy of Doug DeCarlo and ACM)

1.5 Data Acquisition

Designing a realistic body model is a time consuming operation since it requires skilled designer interaction in all stages of the model construction pipeline. Even with dedicated designers and tools (Poser 7 2007), it is almost always impossible to generate one to one correspondence between the real model and the virtual prototype. Since the virtual models have become a very important element of entertainment applications such as games, automatic model construction methods have evolved rapidly. Instead of using designer generated high cost models, 3D data acquisition methods are preferred for rapid and accurate model generation. Aside from many other domains where 3D data acquisition techniques are used, the main objective of this section is to cover data acquisition from a human body surface. Currently, the application area of the 3D data acquisition technique does not just apply to the game industry, but also to the film, sport, fashion and medicine fields. Because of its importance during the last 10 years, development in this field is evolving rapidly.

Recently, different technologies in the market for 3D data acquisition have emerged. Professional human body scanner systems are specialised in body parts such as face, hand, foot and body. Depending on the production area, one of the scanner systems type is preferred to generate an output with optimal quality. For example, the face scanners can acquire high resolution surface information from a small region with texture mapping, while the foot scanner generates rough data but is less costly.

Human body scanner systems are designed with one of the following two main approaches. In the first approach, coloured light patterns are projected on the model. According to the lines' curvature, a surface structure is acquired. In the second approach, a laser light is projected on the model and with a similar procedure surface information is acquired. The first is a low cost approach but in the second, it is possible to acquire very detailed surface information within a resolution of 2 mm. These scanner systems produce 3D point clouds in addition to texture information. By means of the tools provided with the system or by third party applications, the post processing stage takes place to generate the final 3D model. This post processing stage consists of the following steps: Resulting point cloud information filtered from noisy data. Noisy data is produced because of the errors in calibration, the ambient light property of the system environment, and the vibration of the scanned model during the acquisition. Regarding the posture of the subject, the resulting data may contain holes if the cameras could not capture enough data. The hole filling process is another step to produce a reliable complete model. After these steps, the model is divided into cylindrical segments such as arms, legs and torso to have them triangulated. Once the triangulated body model is generated, image processing techniques are used to generate texture coordinates and texture mapping. Finally, recent systems have allowed anthropometric body measurements to be extracted automatically from the scanned data.

1.5.1 Data Acquisition and Reconstruction Pipeline

The scanner uses a laser light stripe (laser triangulation) method for measurements. The principles of this method are shown in Fig. 1.32.

The laser light in combination with a cylindrical lens is used as a light source. A video camera is positioned in a predefined angle to the laser light source. The light line is imaged on the objects which are in the view field of the camera. This line light is deflected by the different heights of the objects.

The angle **W** between the camera and the light source determines the magnitude of the offset and the deflection. The greater the angle **W** means the greater the offset (Fig. 1.32).

The scanning process is completed by moving the laser and camera units over the whole object without vibration. These laser and camera units are moved in a nominal constant speed over the objects for homogeneous data resolution. To get a 360° scan of the objects, several cameras and more than one laser light source are used. In recently used scanners, half of the camera is at the bottom of the laser light source and the other half is at the top, as shown in Fig. 1.33. So, each laser light source has two cameras to scan the hidden areas, as represented in Fig. 1.34.

The acquisition of data from all around the model requires more than one set of laser lights and cameras. A sample organisation of the laser lights and cameras of a human body scanner is represented in Fig. 1.35.

As shown in Fig. 1.34, two scan heads move at the same time along the objects. The speed of the movement determines the resolution of the vertical scanning plane. If it is too fast, then resolution is low but the scan time is shorter.

In Fig. 1.34, details of the scan process are represented with only one laser light source and two cameras. While the scan head moves along the objects, it captures slices. In Fig. 1.34, three slices are represented with blue, red and green lines in sequence. These slices are the laser light line imaged on the object. A rotational angle sensor supplies clock signals to capture different slices while the scan head

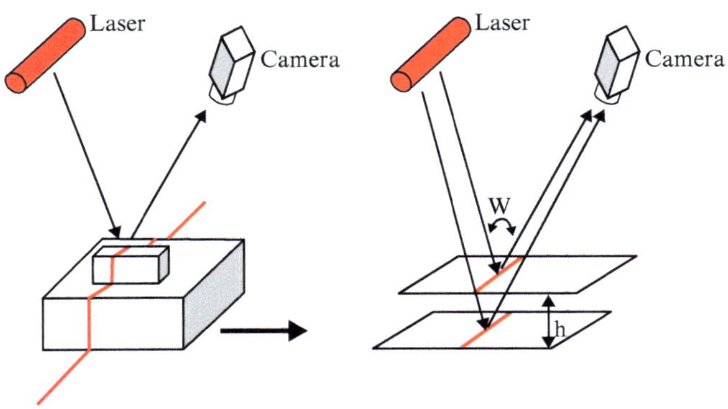

Fig. 1.32 Offset determination and triangulation method

Fig. 1.33 Camera and laser placement

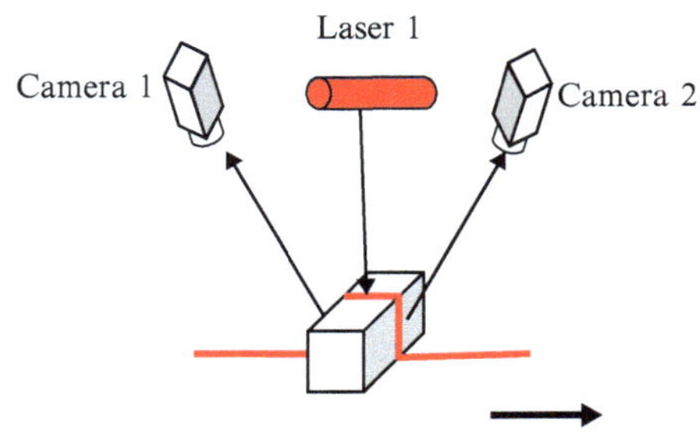

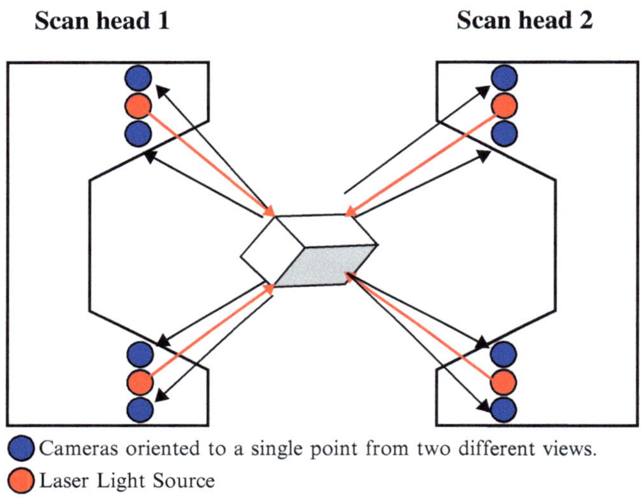

Fig. 1.34 Different scan frames

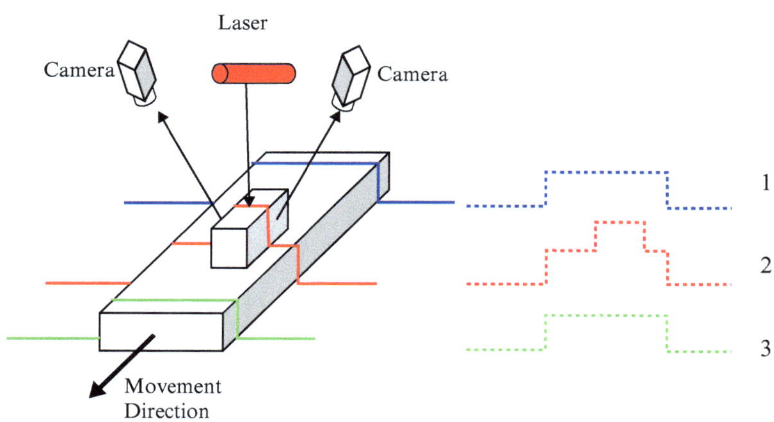

Fig. 1.35 Top view of scan heads with multiple cameras and laser lights

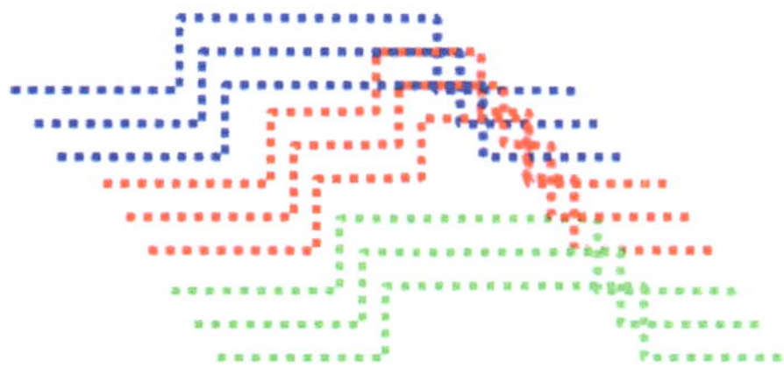

Fig. 1.36 Combined slides

moves along the objects. The movement of the scan head along the object and the captured slices are represented in Fig. 1.36.

Next, the scanner system combines these slices to get the exact representation of the object in an electronic form. The resulting combined slices are represented in Fig. 1.36.

After combining the slices, a point cloud representation of the objects is generated in 3D space. Up to this paragraph, we have described the sequences to generate the point cloud within the human body scanner system. The resulting data (point cloud) is post processed in another system with a special application that may be executed by a standard power computer. With this application, the resulting point cloud data can be triangulated to generate a mesh. The resulting triangulated point cloud data can be stored in standard DXF, OBJ, STL, etc. file formats.

As well as the 3D point cloud data, the scanning system can provide the colour information of each slide. Colour information is provided separately from the point cloud data. Matching the colour information and the point cloud data takes place with the triangulation application described above. During the movement of the scan heads, colour cameras take photos of the objects from different viewpoints. This colour information is generated as the final data along with the point cloud data from the scanner system. Again, in another standard power computer, this colour information is matched with the triangulated point cloud. A special application running on a separate computer first triangulates the point cloud. Next, it applies image processing algorithms on these photos for colour and brightness correction. Then it subtracts the background colour information from the photos. Finally, with special algorithms, this colour information is combined and mapped on the objects. In Fig. 1.37 a sample human body scanner system is represented by a statue in a scan session.

1.5.2 Data Resolution and Data Format

Depending on the scanner system there is a big variation in the resolution of the captured data. Current systems can capture around a million data points from a human body. In the case of laser systems, which can acquire detailed surface information, the surface colour of the subject is very important. If someone wears shiny clothes or has shiny hair, the laser light might not reflect properly, resulting in a shortage of captured data by the cameras. Therefore, the amount of acquired data

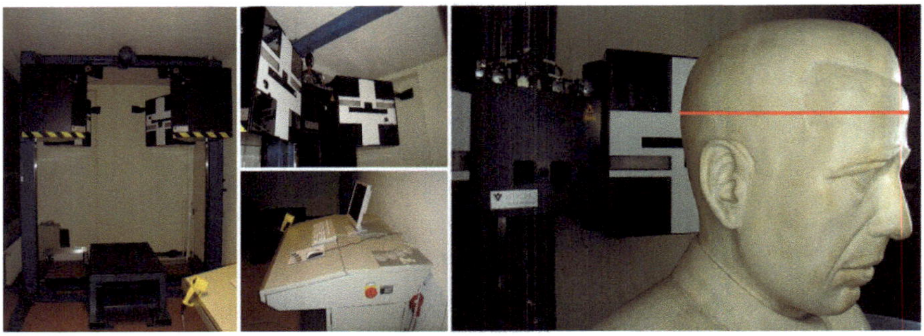

Fig. 1.37 Human body scanning system (Courtesy of MIRAlab Research Laboratory, University of Geneva)

can vary hugely from subject to subject. In most cases, around a million points are acquired which makes it impossible to efficiently visualise it with a standard graphic pipeline. As is represented in Fig. 1.36, the movement of the scan head is very precise, to the millimetre. This results in a huge amount of captured slices where the distance between each slice is represented in millimetres. The distance between consequence points on a single slice is also measured in millimetres. In summary, current 3D body scanner systems can capture and generate one to one virtual representation of a human body.

Generally, each scanner system has its own internal data representation format to store the captured raw data points. Once this data is post processed to generate a single mesh with texture, it can be exported into a standard 3D model file format. Since most of these standard file formats have a text based internal data representation, the size of a file that holds the scanned body model is generally around 100 MB. So, using either binary 3D file formats or reducing the data precision will result in acceptable file sizes.

1.5.3 Scan Data Based Modeling Approaches

The main benefit of the scanned data is the surface detail that is as precise as the scanned subject. It is possible to capture all the surface details along with the skin colour information that is mapped on the resulting mesh. However, the resulting data is a static mesh without any skinning information. For this reason, additional processing stages are required to animate the data. This phase of the process consists of motion adaptation, skeleton adaptation and the skinning stages. Recently, there have been attempts to implement a full automatic pipeline where the scanned model is virtually animated. An earlier approach was carried out by Seo in 2004 (Seo and Magnenat-Thalmann 2004). She used a template body model with predefined feature marks and skinning information. Later this model was registered

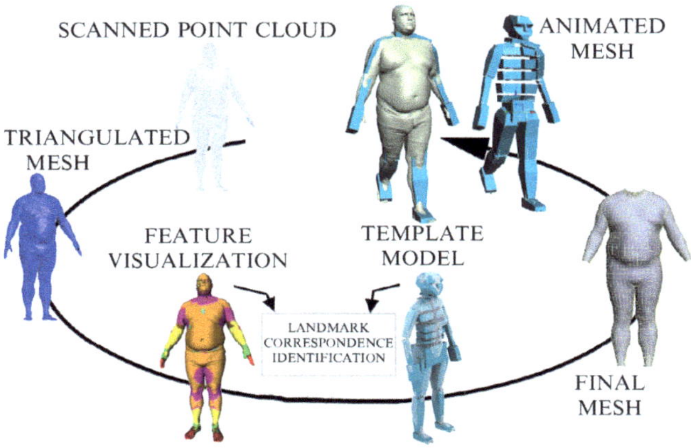

Fig. 1.38 Template based body modeling

on a scanned data to get a similar shape. Since the template model has all the necessary information for animation, the scanned resemblance also has the same information. This process is schematically represented in Fig. 1.38.

References

Azuola F., Badler N., Ho P., Kakadiaris I., Metaxas D., Ting B.: Building anthropometry-based virtual human models, Proceedings of the IMAGE VII conference, IEEE Computer Society, Tuscon, AZ (1994)

Azuola F., Badler N., Hoon T., Wei S.: Sass v.2.1 anthropometric spreadsheet and database for the iris, Department of Computer and Information Science, University of Pennsylvania (1993)

Barr A.: Global and local deformations of solid primitives, SIGGRAPH '84: Proceedings of the 11th annual conference on Computer graphics and interactive techniques, ACM Press, 21–30 (1984)

Blanc C.: Superquadrics A generic implementation of axial procedural deformation techniques, In Graphics Gems, Academic Press, 5, 249–256 (1994)

Borrel P., Rappoport A.: Simple constrained deformations for geometric modeling and interactive design, ACM Trans. Graph., ACM Press, 13, 137–155 (1994)

Chadwick J. E., Haumann D. R., Parent R. E.: Layered construction for deformable animated characters, SIGGRAPH '89: Proceedings of the 16th annual conference on Computer graphics and interactive techniques, ACM Press, 243–252 (1989)

DeCarlo D., Metaxas D., Stone M.: An anthropometric face model using variational techniques, SIGGRAPH '98: Proceedings of the 25th annual conference on Computer graphics and interactive techniques, ACM Press, 67–74 (1998)

Decaudin P.: Geometric deformation by merging a 3D object with a simple shape, Proceedings of Graphics interface '96, 55–60 (1996)

Dooley M.: Anthropometric Modeling Programs – a survey IEEE Comput. Graph. Appl., IEEE Computer Society Press, 2, 17–25 (1982)

Forsey D. R., Bartels R. H.: Hierarchical B-spline refinement, SIGGRAPH '88: Proceedings of the 15th annual conference on Computer graphics and interactive techniques, ACM Press, 205–212 (1988)

Hyun D. E., Yoon S. H., Kim M. S., Jittler B.: Modeling and deformation of arms and legs based on ellipsoidal sweeping. In PG '03: Proceedings of the 11th pacific conference on Computer graphics and applications, IEEE Computer Society, 204–212 (2003)

Kasap M., Magnenat-Thalmann N.: Parameterized human body model for real-time applications, CW '07 International conference on Cyberworlds, IEEE Computer Society, 160–167 (2007)

Lamousin H. J., Jr., Waggenspack W. N.: NURBS-based free-form deformations, IEEE Comput. Graph. Appl., IEEE Computer Society Press, 14, 59–65 (1994)

Larboulette C., Cani M., Arnaldi B.: Dynamic skinning: adding real-time dynamic effects to an existing character animation SCCG '05: Proceedings of the 21st spring conference on Computer graphics, ACM Press, 87–93 (2005)

Magnenat-Thalmann N., Laperrière R., Thalmann D.: Joint-dependent local deformations for hand animation and object grasping, Proceedings on Graphics interface '88, Canadian Information Processing Society, 26–33 (1988)

Magnenat-Thalmann N., Thalmann D.: The Direction of Synthetic Actors in the Film Rendez-vous à Montréal, IEEE Computer Graphics and Applications, 7, 9-19 (1987)

Magnenat-Thalmann N. (Producer), Thalmann D.: Rendez-vous à Montréal. International Telefilm, Ltd., Montreal, Canada (1987)

Nedel L., Thalmann D.: Modeling and deformation of the human body using an anatomically-based approach, CA '98: Proceedings of the Computer animation, IEEE Computer Society, 34 (1998)

Poser 7, http://www.e-frontier.com. Accessed 15 March 2007 (2007)

Pratscher M., Coleman P., Laszlo J., Singh K.: Outside-in anatomy based character rigging. In SCA '05: Proceedings of the 2005 ACM SIGGRAPH/Eurographics symposium on Computer animation, ACM Press, 329–338 (2005)

Requicha H.: Solid Modeling: A Historical Summary and Contemporary Assessment Computer Graphics and Applications, IEEE, 2, 9–24 (1982)

Scheepers F., Parent R. E., Carlson W. E., May S. F.: Anatomy-based modeling of the human musculature, SIGGRAPH '97: Proceedings of the 24th annual conference on Computer graphics and interactive techniques, ACM Press/Addison-Wesley Publishing Co., 163–172 (1997)

Sederberg T. W., Parry S. R.: Free-form deformation of solid geometric models, SIGGRAPH '86: Proceedings of the 13th annual conference on Computer graphics and interactive techniques, ACM Press, 151–160 (1986)

Seo H., Magnenat-Thalmann N.: An example-based approach to human body manipulation Graph. Models, Academic Press Professional, Inc., 66, 1–23 (2004)

Shen J., Magnenat-Thalmann N., Thalmann D.: Human skin deformation from cross-sections computer graphics Int. '94 (1994)

Singh K., Fiume E.: Wires: a geometric deformation technique, SIGGRAPH '98: Proceedings of the 25th annual conference on Computer graphics and interactive techniques, ACM Press, 405–414 (1998)

Steindler A.: "Kinesiology of the Human Body", Charles C. Thomas Publisher, Springfield Illinois (1955)

Teran J., Sifakis E., Blemker S. S., Ng-Thow-Hing V., Lau C., Fedkiw R.: Creating and simulating skeletal, muscle from the visible human data set, IEEE Transactions on Visualization and Computer Graphics, IEEE Educational Activities Department, 11, 317–328 (2005)

Terzopoulos D., Platt J., Barr A., Fleischer K.: Elastically deformable models, SIGGRAPH '87: Proceedings of the 14th annual conference on Computer graphics and interactive techniques, ACM, 205–214 (1987)

Wilhelms J.: Modeling Animals with Bones, Muscles, and Skin, Technical Report: UCSC-CRL-95-01, University of California at Santa Cruz (1995)

Chapter 2
Character Based Adaptation

Abstract This chapter reviews the techniques that are required for efficiently and accurately animate virtual human models. The techniques described here enable one to tailor the animation to specific subjects, including their shape, and weight characteristics. These animations can then be used to produce virtual catwalks, which in turn can be used as a basis for a virtual try on application.

2.1 Introduction

Virtual characters are of great interest for the computer graphics community. Generate pictures that look human, move human and behave human is a challenging problem, stemming lots of different issues that must be solved depending on the application and context of the targeted application. Thus, many approaches were proposed already for addressing the technical difficulties that one encounters when following this path. The directions of research dealing with this particular topic are many. Modeling, animation and rendering are the main aspects that were investigated, and as soon as a virtual human appears on a screen, this field of research becomes closely linked with other sciences such as cognitive, psychological and social sciences. This chapter, however, only deals with character animation, and more specifically with motion adaptation as it is a wide enough topic by itself, without considering aspects such as how an audience perceives the animation or the feeling that is triggered by such or such stimuli.

2.1.1 Character Animation

The general principle for animating a virtual 3D character – whatever it looks like – is as follows. First of all the character is given an underlying skeleton with a hierarchical structure (Fig. 2.1 which is the object that drives the animation. Because of its hierarchical formulation (i.e. each limb is placed with respect to the limb

N. Magnenat-Thalmann (ed.), *Modeling and Simulating Bodies and Garments*,
DOI 10.1007/978-1-84996-263-6_2, © Springer-Verlag London Limited 2010

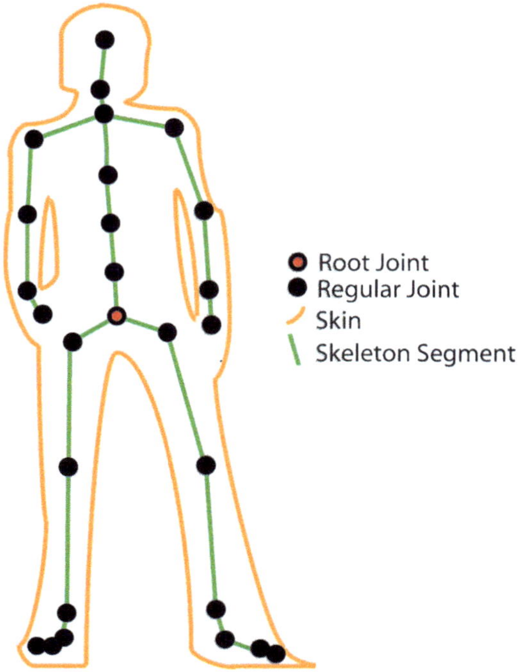

Fig. 2.1 Principle of a character animation. The skeleton (in *green*) is first placed in the 3D space thanks to the transformation of a root joint. The skeleton is then put in the right pose by rotating its other joints, and finally the skin (in *orange*) is deformed according to the skeleton

onto which it is attached), all the joints rotations and segments offsets must be computed, along with one unique root transformation used for placing the skeleton in space. This approach can be seen as placing the character at its correct location and then adapt its pose for the current frame. It has many benefits, such as the possibility to easily edit the skeleton pose in order to make it match a desired configuration by simply rotating the joints (because of the hierarchical formulation, rotating the shoulder joint moves the entire arm), or the fact that a given animation can be applied on various skeletons without having to re-compute the rotation of all the joints. The drawbacks – tightly linked to the benefits – are that because it exists no explicit relationship between an animation and the sizes of a skeleton, a motion can be directly applied on only one skeleton and one must adapt – or retarget – the motion before applying it on another skeleton. This problem can be illustrated as follows: two characters with different sizes and shapes (for instance one tall and on small), while walking, do not travel the same distance when they perform the exact same number of steps. But because the global location of a skeleton is recorded once and for all when the animation is created, the global location of the root joint of the animation does not match the

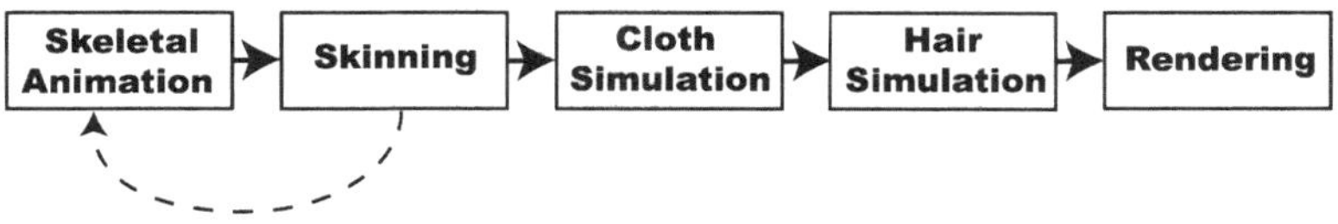

Fig. 2.2 The character animation process. From an existing skeletal animation, a skin is attached to the skeleton bones. In case the skin conflicts with the animation (because of self penetrations for instance) then the animation is modified (*dashed arrow*). Once a satisfying character animation is obtained, other elements can be added such as cloth simulation or hair. Eventually, the animation is rendered either in real-time or offline

new length of the limbs, and the character has its feet sliding on the ground, if not penetrating it or floating in the air.

Once the underlying skeleton is animated, the character is given a virtual skin: this is the skinning stage (Fig. 2.2). A virtual skin is a 3D mesh attached to the skeleton in such a way that it follows the skeleton animation. The attachment process consists of defining a relationship between each vertex of the skin and a subset of bones from the skeleton so that the skin follows the motion of the skeleton in a sound and realistic manner. Even if the skinning attachment is done very carefully by skilled animators, it can also yield to various unpleasant visual artifacts which are usually corrected afterwards by hand. Basically, the same adaptation issues that appear for the skeleton have their skin equivalent. For instance, if the skeleton animation was created with a slim morphology in mind, applying it to a fat character makes the body penetrate itself because the actual girth of each limb is now much larger.

Finally, once a nice looking skinned character is obtained, additional features are added: cloth, hair and more. However, because this third phase is out of the scope of this chapter, it will be discussed later. A conceptual view of this animation process can be seen on Fig. 2.2.

2.2 Previous Works

Early works (Popovic and Witkin 1995; Bruderlin and Williams 1995) tackled the problem of editing an existing animation clip by using interpolation and wavelet decomposition. Gleicher (1997) proposed an algorithm based on spacetime optimization (Witkin and Kass 1988) for the same purpose. He was the first one to introduce the notion of adaptation – or retargeting – for mapping an existing motion to a new character (Gleicher 1998). His method consists of defining characteristics of the motion that the user wants to keep as a set of constraints to be solved by a spacetime optimization algorithm. The optimization algorithm computes an adapted motion that re-establishes the constraints while preserving the characteristics of the original motion.

Popovic (Popovic and Witkin 1999; Popovic 2000) again used spacetime optimization for correcting the physical behavior of a motion clip. His approach used a simplified version of the character to reduce the complexity of the problem. Tak (Tak and Ko 2005) used a slightly different approach to address the same issue. A Kalman filter estimates the state of the character at a given frame, and the pose is then optimized according to constraints defined by the designer. As the optimization is performed on a single frame instead of the whole sequence, it performs much faster than the previous approaches. Abe (Abe et al. 2006) revisited the spacetime optimization approach. No simplification of the skeleton is required, and an interpolation scheme enables to achieve real-time performances. Shin (Shin et al. 2003) used closed-form method and hierarchical displacement maps to influence the physical properties of a motion.

Choi and Ko (2000) used inverse rate control to perform a retargeting in real-time. Their algorithm is able to enforce several constraints while adapting a motion to a new character.

Lee and Shin (1999) introduced the use of Inverse Kinematics (IK) for editing motion while Tolani (Tolani et al. 2000) investigated how to reach real-time performances for moving the arm or leg of a virtual character through an analytical solution for a limb with 7 degrees of freedom (DoF). Boulic (Boulic et al. 2003; Baerlocher and Boulic 2003) extended the classical IK algorithms to include the concept of priorities among the constraints. The higher priority constraint is enforced first, and the search space is then projected onto the subspace that satisfies the first constraint.

Preventing collisions or penetration with the environment and/or with the character itself has also been investigated by the community. Applying a motion to a body that it does not match produces interpenetration between objects in case of a virtual environment, while in the case of real robots it might turn out to be much more problematic, as it can yield to damage equipment.

Zhao and Badler (1994) were among the first to address this issue. They introduced the concept of sensors attached to the body which monitor the collisions occurrence. For a set of collision primitive (ellipsoids, half-spaces and cylindrical tubes) they defined potential functions, which are positive inside the collision volumes only. In case a positive potential is detected, an IK step takes place to minimize the potential of the sensor.

This concept of sensor was later integrated in a framework dedicated to virtual humans by Boulic et al. (1997). He and others improved this approach by coupling it with prioritized IK. Instead of using potential fields, they defined a damping volume around the collision primitives (Peinado et al. 2005), which smoothly prevents the observers (an entity analog to a sensor) from colliding with the surrounding environment or itself (Peinado et al. 2007). Once coupled with a postural control engine (Peinado et al. 2006), which animates the character from mocap data, it is thus possible to control an avatar in real-time with collision avoidance. Kuffner et al. (2002) proposed to use sets of threshold distance between specific points on the body to monitor and prevent self collision. As in the previously mentioned approaches, the potential collisions are detected before they actually happen, and are thus prevented rather than corrected. Jeong and Lee (2000) correct rather than prevent such artifacts, in case the animation is applied to a character slightly different from the capture subject. They also use collision volumes attached to the skeleton so that the character shape is taken into account and correct the penetration using numerical IK.

More recently, Chai and Hodgins (2007) used a statistical model learned from example motions to bind the motion adaptation process. By learning what is possible or not, the system thus only generates natural looking motions.

2.3 A Footskate Removal Method for Simplified Characters

VR applications are quite different from entertainment productions. Indeed, VR aims at immersing a user in a real time environment as similar as possible to reality. Thus these applications are usually highly demanding in terms of performances. To meet these requirements, most labs have built their own VR platforms (Ponder et al. 2003; Website VR Juggler 2008) which allow to re-use previously developed components. These frameworks are optimized to ensure maximum performances at runtime, and most of the models assume numerous simplifications in order to allow for rich environments. For instance, VHD++ developed jointly by MIRALab, University of Geneva and VRLab, EPFL allows to create virtual characters animations, thus enabling the creation of advanced application, such as virtual try on. For such application, the user gives his/her dimensions to the system which then generates an avatar according to the specifications. Once the avatar is created, its size must remain constant so that it resembles the user. This requirement forbids the use of the method proposed by (Kovar et al. 2002). Moreover, VR developers rarely focus on side artifacts and usually prefer to concentrate on the final user experience, which prevents them from implementing complex methods for little benefits. The method we propose here complies with the two previous statements in the sense that it can accommodate rigid skeletons and is very easy to implement. Thus it can be added with only little time and effort to an existing VR framework.

The method can be summarized as follows: first foot plants are estimated, i.e. when should each foot be planted on the ground. Unlike most of the other approaches, our algorithm does not constrain the *location* where a foot is planted, but rather the *frame* at which this should happen. This way, the motion itself remains as close as possible to the original, only the path followed by the character is subject to a scale.

The next stage is divided into two separate processes. A first treatment corrects the character's motion along the horizontal axis, and a second one adapts its vertical displacement. This choice was motivated by the observation that in most VR applications, the feet of the character remain rigid throughout the animations. This happens because the feet are attached to only one joint, again for optimization reasons. Thus, as the skin is not deformed accurately, the feet will somewhat penetrate the ground regardless of the retargeting process applied. To correct this, our method accurately plant the feet where they should be in the horizontal plane, while in the vertical direction it minimizes the distance between the ground and the planted foot.

2.3.1 *Feet Motion Analysis*

Depending on the quality of a motion clip, it can be quite tricky to estimate how and when to plant a foot. If the motion is perfect, it should be enough to simply observe that a foot remaining static may be planted. However, feet are rarely motionless. Moreover most of the clips that are repeatedly used in reality are far from perfect and therefore such a simple criterion is insufficient. Previous works focused on proximity rules to extract the planting (Bindiganavale and Badler 1998), k-nearest neighbors classifier (Ikemoto et al. 2006) or adaptive threshold imposed on the location and velocity of the feet (Glardon et al. 2006).

All the above mentioned approaches require some human interaction to perform the estimation: even (Glardon et al. 2006) requires to at least specify the kind of motion being performed. As we mentioned previously, our goal is to discard this interaction stage. Instead, we applied a two steps estimation taking the root translation and foot vertices into account. The first step finds out which foot should be planted while the second one refines which part of the sole should remain static.

This is achieved by first extracting from the skin mesh the vertices for which the speed has to be calculated. We then isolate the vertices belonging to the feet by using the skin attachment data. Finally, we remove the ones for which the normal is not pointing downward, which leaves us with the sole. For clarity reasons, we will use t to designate a frame index or a time interval, the unit corresponding to the actual time elapsed between two animation frames.

2.3.1.1 Foot Selection

Given the original root translation ΔR_t from time t to $t + 1$ and v_i the vertex which is planted at frame t, we estimate which foot must remain planted at frame $t + 1$ by considering the motion $\Delta R'_t$ for which the sole vertex v_j remains planted during the next animation frame. By planting a vertex at time t, we mean that its global coordinates remain constant during the time interval $[t - 0.5, t + 0.5]$. $\Delta R'_t$ can thus simply be expressed as:

$$\Delta R'_t = o(\upsilon_i, t) - o(\upsilon_i, t+\delta) + o(\upsilon_j, t+\delta) - o(\upsilon_j, t+1)$$

$o(v_i, t)$ being the offset at frame t of vertex v_i from the root, in world coordinates (Fig. 2.3). For this estimation, we take $\delta = 0.5$ and $o(v_i, t + \delta)$ is calculated by linear interpolation between t and $t + 1$.

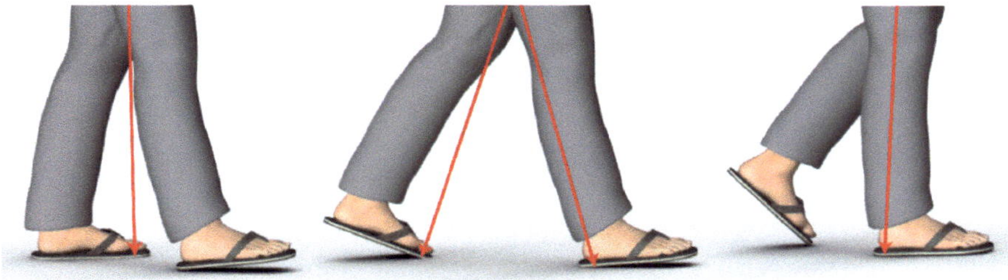

Fig. 2.3 Offsets for foot skating removal. On the left, vertex v_i is planted, and remains so until $t + \delta$. At that time, vertex v_j becomes planted until $t + 1$, i.e. the next frame. For clarity reason, more than one frame elapsed between the poses displayed on this figure

Once we calculated $\Delta R'_t$ for all the sole vertices, we designate as static the vertex that maximizes the dot product p:

$$p = \frac{\Delta R_t}{\|\Delta R_t\|} \cdot \frac{\Delta R'_t}{\|\Delta R'_t\|}$$

Indeed, a higher value of this dot product means that if v_j is static at frame $t + 1$, the displacement induced will resemble more the original root motion. We discard the magnitude of the vector because we are interested in *where* the character is going and not *how far away* it goes.

2.3.1.2 Vertex Selection

The dot product criterion robustly tells us which foot must be planted. However, the actual vertex picked by this algorithm can sometimes be jerky, e.g. jump from the foot tip to the heel. The reason is that we picked the vertex which keeps the motion as close as possible to the original one, possibly keeping a bit of skating on its way. In order to overcome this issue, we add a second selection process applied on the vertices of the planted foot only. This second process uses the *speed* of the vertices in order to pick the right one. Indeed, if the original motion is not too bad, then the vertex which must be static at a given frame is most likely to be the one moving the less. The speed of each vertex is first smoothed along several frames in order to remove some of the data noise (in our experiments, five frames appeared to be a good compromise). Second, the least moving vertex is chosen as the static one. The result of this selection over a foot step can be seen on Fig. 2.4.

We previously assumed that the static vertex in the previous frame must be known in order to estimate the one in the current frame. So for the first frame of the animation, we just use the speed criterion. One could think that the detection would

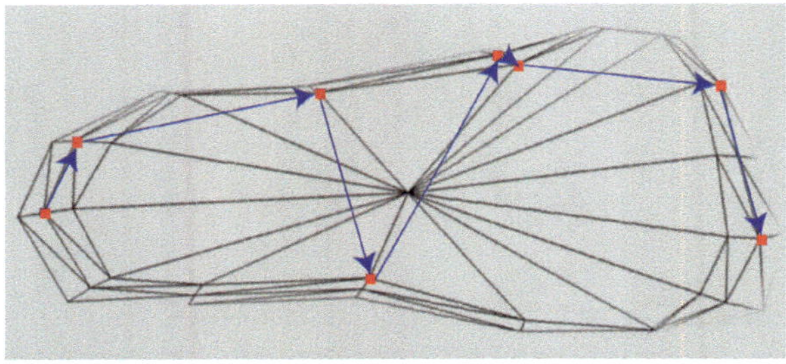

Fig. 2.4 View of the trajectory of the least moving point over the sole during one foot step. In black is a wire frame view of the sole of the character, in red are the vertices selected during the step, and eventually the blue arrows show the transitions between each point

be less accurate because of this; however we did not witness any setback during our experiments.

This algorithm has proven to be quite efficient on the catwalk animations we tried it on. It is even possible to discard the dot product phase of the algorithm but we noticed that this stage of the process significantly improved the robustness of the detection by accurately tagging which foot must be planted. If the original animation clip is too bad, our algorithm may fail to figure out which vertex should be planted. In this case, one still has the possibility to manually label the vertices (or correct the output of the algorithm), as it is the case for all the previous motion retargeting methods. However, during our tests, this only happened on complex dance motions, for which it was hard even for the human eye to figure out which foot should be planted or not.

2.4 Root Translation Correction

The retargeting is split into two phases, namely horizontal and vertical corrections. The horizontal correction introduces a drift of the character over the animation range in order to remove the foot skating, while the vertical processing aims at minimizing the distance of the static vertices from the floor.

These two separate steps use completely different approaches, which are outlined in the next section.

2.4.1 Horizontal Correction

In order to calculate the corrected horizontal translation of the root joint between two frames, once again we use the motion of the vertices. In the previous section, we made the assumption that a static vertex remains so during a time interval of at

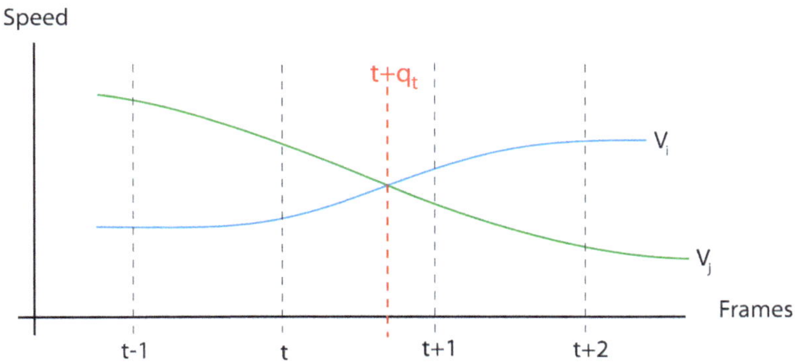

Fig. 2.5 A conceptual view of the velocity estimation performed in order to determinate the exact instant of the weight transfer between two fixed points

least one frame, centered on the current time instant. However, due to the low sampling of the motion data which is often no more than 25 Hz, this assumption cannot be retained for the actual displacement of the root joint. Thus, we estimate when the transition between two static vertices should happen, again using their speed. As we stated that the vertex with the less speed should remain static, we estimate the exact time instant between two frames when the transfer should occur.

For doing so, we approximate the speed of each vertex as follows: first the speed of the current and next static vertices v_i and v_j are calculated for frames $t - 1$, t, $t + 1$ and $t + 2$. These velocities are then plotted in 2D and approximated using a Catmull-Rom spline (Catmull and Rom 1974) which yields to two parametric curves $V_i(q)$ and $V_j(q)$, $q \in [0, 1]$, as depicted on Fig. 2.5. Eventually, the particular value q_t corresponding to the cross between v_i and v_j is calculated by solving the cubic equation $V_i(q) = V_j(q)$, which we did using the approach proposed by Nickalls (1993).

Now that the exact time $t + q_t$ when the weight transfer occurs is known, the actual position of the vertices at this instant is to be calculated. For doing so, the trajectory of the points between t and $t + 1$ is first approximated using again a Catmull-Rom spline. The parametric location t_1 and t_2 of the points over these curves is given by their approximated speeds as follows:

$$t_i = \frac{\int_t^{t+qt} V_i(q)dq}{\int_t^{t+1} V_i(q)dq}, i = 1,2$$

Having the two offsets $o(v_i, t + q_t)$ and $o(v_j, t + q_t)$, enables us to calculate the new root displacement between frames t and $t + 1$ (Fig. 2.6).

The translation computed during this step is valid only if the feet deform in a realistic way which – to our experience – they seldom do. Often they remain rigid and this creates a bad vertical translation while the weight is transferred from the

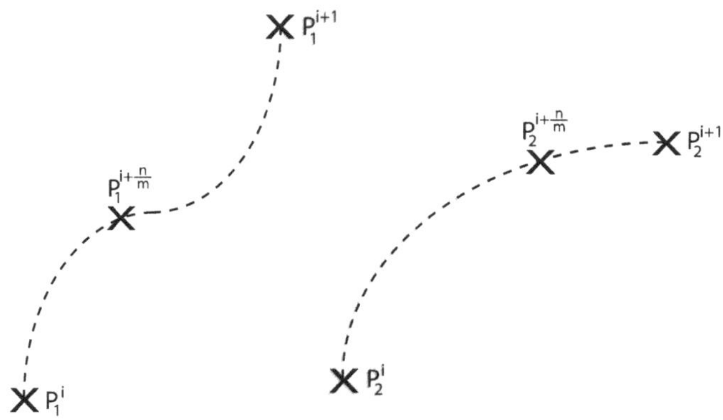

Fig. 2.6 This figure illustrates the trajectory estimate that is performed between the points at frame i and i + 1. m samples are calculated, and the nth one is kept for the later calculation of the root translation

heel to the toe during a foot step. This is the reason why, as stated previously, the calculated root translation is only applied on the horizontal directions, as follows:

$$\Delta R_t^{horizontal} = P.\Delta R_t'$$

P being a 3D to 2D projection matrix.

2.4.2 Vertical Correction

The horizontal correction introduces some drift of the character compared to the original animation. This effect is desired as it removes the foot skating. However, in the vertical direction, no drift should take place otherwise the body will soon be walking in the floor or in the air. We do not want either to change the legs configuration for enforcing the correct height of the foot sole because we want to remain as close as possible from the original animation of the limbs. Moreover, strictly enforcing the height of the static vertices to be zero would lead to cumbersome configurations of the legs in order to cope with the rigidity of the feet (remember that the feet seldom deform in VR applications) thus introducing ugly artifacts.

Instead, we chose to act on the root joint translation only, by minimizing the height of the static vertices over the animation. Thus, a little bit of penetration will remain afterwards, which is the price to pay if the feet are rigid and if we do not want to drastically change the look of the animation.

We calculate a single offset and a scale to be applied to the root height trajectory so that static vertices remain as close as possible from the ground throughout the animation, as shown on Fig. 2.7.

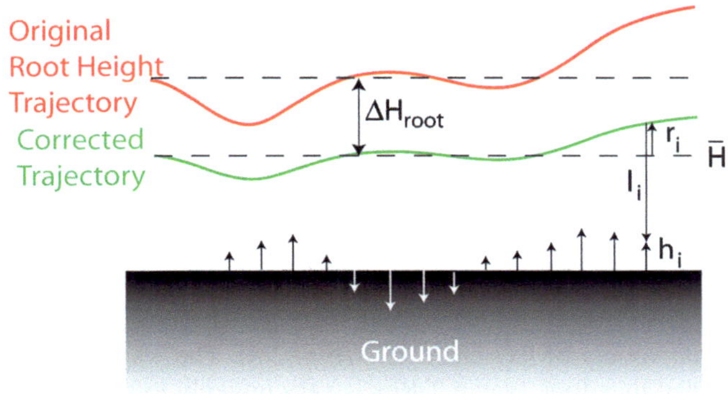

Fig. 2.7 Scaling of the root joint height

It is quite trivial to calculate the offset to be applied to the root trajectory: if we consider the height h_t in world coordinates of each static point, then the root offset ΔH is simply:

$$\Delta H = -\sum_{t=0}^{N-1} \frac{h_t}{N}$$

N being the number of frames of the animation.

Once this offset is applied to the root trajectory, the mean of the static vertices height is thus zero. However, they still oscillate above and underneath the ground during the animation. This oscillation will be minimized by the calculation of the scaling factor α.

If we consider $\overline{H}$ to be the average root height over the animation, then for each frame its actual height H_t can be written as an offset r_t from this mean value: $H_t = \overline{H} + r_t$. The variance σ^2 of the static points heights can be expressed in terms of the root average height $\overline{H}$, the scaling factor α and the relative height l_t of the fixed vertex with respect to the root as follow:

$$N\alpha^2 = \sum_{t=0}^{N-1} h_t^2 = \sum_{t=0}^{N-1} (\overline{H} + \alpha r_t + l_t)^2$$

This variance is to be minimized by the scaling factor α, and fortunately this is equivalent to finding the root of a simple second order equation with only one unknown, α. Indeed:

$$N\alpha^2 = \alpha^2 \sum_{t=0}^{N-1} r_t^2 + 2\alpha \sum_{t=0}^{N-1} (r_t \cdot (\overline{H} + l_t)) + \sum_{t=0}^{N-1} (\overline{H} + l_t)^2$$

As σ^2 and N are always positive, the minimal variance is given by:

$$\alpha = -\frac{\sum_{t=0}^{N-1} r_t \bullet (\overline{H} + l_t)}{\sum_{t=0}^{N-1} r_t^2}$$

2.5 Character Movements Adaptation

2.5.1 Introduction

It exists a wide variety of CG characters (Fig. 2.8). The way they move strongly depends on what they look like: a T-Rex is very unlikely to walk the same way as a fashion model. Thus, when an animation clip is applied to a specific character it should be adapted so that it better match its particular features. For instance, self penetrations should be taken care of otherwise the limbs of the character will penetrate its body. Also, the gait should be adapted so that the motion matches the shape; otherwise an observer will know that something is wrong, even though he or she is not quite able to say what.

One of the most successful approaches for modifying an existing animation is to use a global optimization algorithm in order to do the job. It has been used by various works (Gleicher 1998; Popovic and Witkin 1999; Shin et al. 2003) to address several aspects of the problem, such as foot plant enforcement, constraints compliance and physical properties of the motion. This approach uses a global optimization algorithm in order to modify the entire motion clip in one pass, unlike a per frame approach which would deal with each frame individually. The main advantage of the global approach compared to the local one is that it is possible to introduce a continuity criterion in the adaptation process, thus ensuring a smooth animation. Another benefit is that it is possible to address problems which require that several frames are taken into account in order to adapt a single frame.

One might be tempted to work directly with the recorded animation trajectories, and to modify them so that such or such criterion is satisfied. This has proven to be a bad idea for several reasons. First of all, these curves feature high frequencies coming from the actual character motion, which are of great importance for the

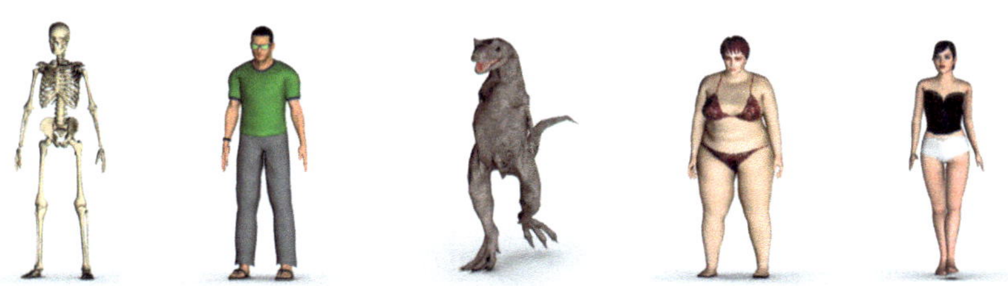

Fig. 2.8 A few example of 3D characters. From left to right a human skeleton, an athletic man, a T-Rex, a plump lady and a skinny lady

natural look of the movement. These frequencies must be kept otherwise the adapted motion will be degraded much. Thus working directly with these curves will introduce big discontinuities in the optimization which would most certainly trap the optimizer in local minima. Second, depending on how the motion data is stored, it might take an extra step to extract the animation curves for each degree of freedom. If the skeleton rotations are stored using quaternion for instance, they will have to be converted to Euler angles first to be usable in the optimizer. Hence it is best to add an extra animation layer coming from the optimizer rather than dealing with the animation curves themselves.

The setup of the adaptation algorithm starts by defining the degrees of freedom (DoF) available to the optimizer. Each DoF will allow the algorithm to modify the orientation of one of the skeleton joint along a given axis. A typical animation is several hundreds of frames long, which would spawn hundreds of variables (one per frame) per DoF. A typical way to reduce the number of variables is to use control points of spline curves instead of their actual values. This approach also has the advantage to prevent the optimizer from adding high frequencies to the motion, which are very noticeable and would make the final motion less realistic. The drawback is that the control points must be carefully chosen as the final result is quite dependent on them. In our experiments, we noticed that a good way to place the control points is to roughly estimate where the minima and maxima of the corrections should be, and to place control points at these particular time instants.

The general problem of adapting a motion can be formulated as follows:

$$\begin{aligned} &\min_{x \in \mathbb{R}^n} f(x) \\ &s.t. x^l \leq x \leq x^u \\ &\quad g_j(x) \leq 0, j \in I^n \\ &\quad h_k(x) = 0, k \in I^{ne} \end{aligned}$$

with x the vector of unknown, f the function to minimize,[1] x^l and x^u the lower and upper bounds of the variables, g_j the set of inequality constraints (would they be linear or not) and h_j the set of equality constraints.

In the motion adaptation process, x will be formed by the set of DoFs available, f will be the quantity to be minimized (e.g. difference from the original motion) while g and h are used to make sure that some constraints are kept during the adaptation process (e.g. keep the planted foot on the ground). This works well if the starting point of the process complies with the constraints. In case the starting point does not comply with all the constraints, then the optimizer must generate a new starting point which can sometimes turn out to be very difficult to do.

[1] There could be more than one function to minimize, however this was left aside here for the sake of simplicity.

We rather choose to use penalty functions in order to express the constraints. This works well for inequality constraints if the weights associated with each function are properly defined. Equality constraints are more difficult to enforce due to the limitation they impose on the variables. The optimization becomes:

$$\min_{x\in\mathbb{R}^n} \alpha f(x) + \sum_j \beta_j p_j(x) + \sum_k \gamma_k h_k(x), j \in I^n, k \in I^{ne}$$

$$p_j(x) = \begin{cases} g_j(x) & \text{if } g_j(x) \geq 0 \\ 0 & \text{otherwise} \end{cases}$$

The variables bounds can simply be enforced by clamping the variables to their min and max values.

Even though well defined, large systems are usually quite difficult to deal with. The high number of variables makes it difficult for the algorithm to figure out where to look for the optimal solution. Numerous valleys exhibiting local minima might trap the search, while peaks may prevent the algorithm from searching in all the solution space. It exists a way to break down a complex optimization into smaller, easier pieces called block coordinates descent (Betts and Smith 2001; Cohen 1992; Liu et al. 2006). This approach assigns sets of variables which will be fixed while the other variables are being optimized. It works well if the variables are somewhat disjoint from each other, while it might have difficulties in finding the true minimum if the variables are too much correlated. Fortunately, the individual motion of a character's limbs is well separated from limb to limb. Thus, an approach similar to block coordinate descent was adopted and each limb is adapted separately as shown on Fig. 2.9.

Breaking the problem into smaller pieces not only makes the convergence faster, but it also drastically reduces the computation time. Indeed, because the character motion is pre-recorded, it is hard to find an analytic formulation for the derivatives of the motion. The derivatives of the motion are estimated through finite difference thus leading to a $O(n^2)$ calculation at each step of the optimization, n being the number of free variables.

2.5.2 Skeleton Design

In order to keep the adaptation framework as general as possible, we choose to use a character studio's Biped hierarchy (Fig. 2.10) which has 30 joints and 29 bones. The joints are not constrained, thus they can freely rotate around their axis and possibly go further than a real human could. This may be a problem when adding corrections on top of the existing rotations because there is no direct way to detect that a joint went further than what it can normally do. Fortunately we did not notice such issue as long as the problem is well stated.

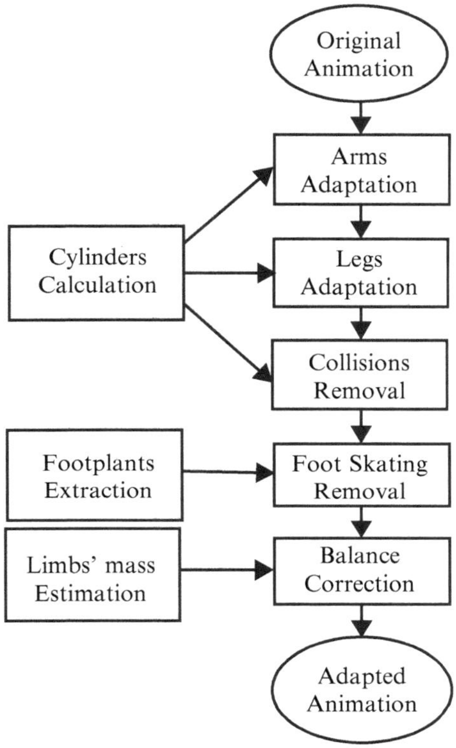

Fig. 2.9 Conceptual representation of the motion adaptation process

2.5.2.1 Limbs Simplification

The adaptation does not have to completely satisfy the penetration constraints, because for this the skin itself should deform in a physical way. Thus, instead of calculating the actual penetration distance between the limbs, an approximate value will be computed and used in subsequent calculations. For doing so, we first match one cylinder per joint of the skeleton. To make each cylinder better reflect the actual volume of the limb, we will use the average distance of the mesh vertices from the bone as radius for the cylinder.

The calculation of each average distance is done by first calculating the covariance matrix $\sum_i$ for each limb, as follows:

$$\Sigma_i = \sum_j \begin{pmatrix} x_j^2 & x_j y_j & x_j z_j \\ x_j y_j & y_j^2 & y_j z_j \\ x_j z_j & y_j z_j & z_j^2 \end{pmatrix} \quad j \in I_i^{bm}$$

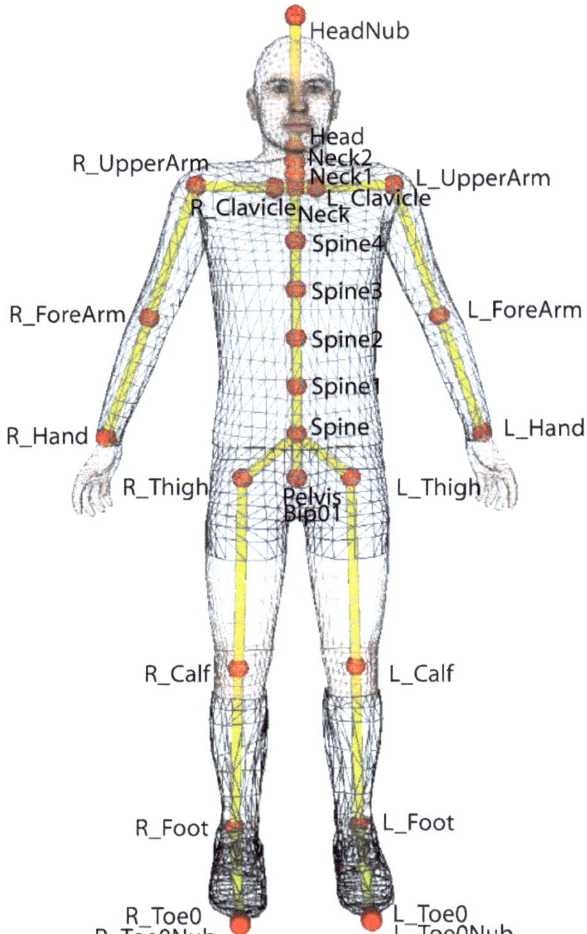

Fig. 2.10 The biped hierarchy

Here x_j, y_j and z_j are the coordinates of vertex j. I^{bm}_i is the set of vertices to be considered for that particular cylinder. The mean of the vertices coordinates was subtracted from the set of vertices beforehand so that the data set is centered on 0.

Next, the eigenvectors and eigenvalues are calculated for each matrix (Press et al. 1992). Most likely, the first eigenvalue and eigenvector corresponds to the direction of the bone, the two remaining ones to the actual radius of the cylinder. This can be confirmed by discarding the eigenvector which gives the greatest dot product with the bone direction vector. Eventually, the radius of a cylinder can be taken as the average of the two remaining eigenvalues. An example of the generated cylinders can be seen on Fig. 2.11.

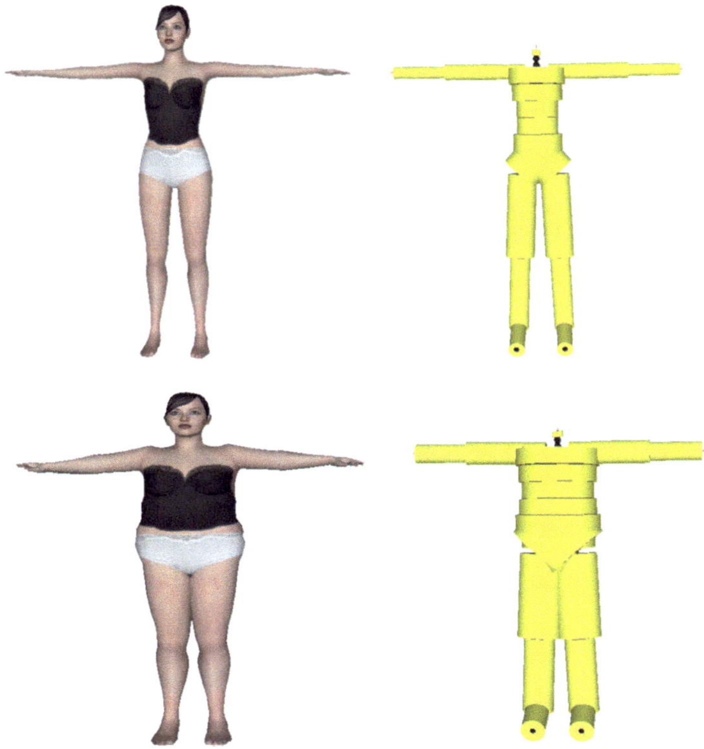

Fig. 2.11 Two virtual characters (*left*) and their cylinders counterparts (*right*)

2.5.2.2 Vertex/Cylinder Allocation

The cylinders layout is predefined so that it neatly fits the body shape (Fig. 2.13). To know which vertex will contribute to a particular cylinder we proceed as follows: first we use the skinning data to find out a rough location over the body, as follows:

$$C_i = Max\left(w_{i1},.,w_{in}\right)$$

With c_i the index of the cylinder to which the vertex number i might contribute, w_{ij} the weight of influence of bone number j to vertex number i and n the number of bones influencing vertex i.

Because vertex i might as well contribute to cylinder c_i as one of its neighbors, we orthogonally project the vertex onto the axis of c_i but also onto the axis of its two neighboring segments. The cylinder onto which the orthogonal projection falls is retained as cylinder associated with vertex i.

2.5.2.3 Penetration Calculation

The use of cylinders allowed us to speed up the process of detecting penetrations compared to a lower level approach such as collision detection on the skin mesh. However, it is not trivial to compute the penetration of a cylinder with a fixed length, and thus a fast and robust algorithm is given here. First, the minimal distance between the two lines supporting the cylinders is calculated. Each line is defined by a point and vector, as illustrated on Fig. 2.12. The minimal distance between these two lines can be retrieved by calculating two points: $P(s) = P_0 + s_c\vec{u}$ and $Q(t) = Q_0 + t_c\vec{v}$ which define the vector $\vec{w}_c$ perpendicular to both lines as follows:

$$
\begin{aligned}
a &= \vec{u}\cdot\vec{u} \\
b &= \vec{u}\cdot\vec{v} \\
c &= \vec{v}\cdot\vec{v} \\
d &= \vec{u}\cdot\vec{w}_0 \\
e &= \vec{v}\cdot\vec{w}_0 \\
s_c &= \frac{be - cd}{ac - b^2} \\
t_c &= \frac{ad - bd}{ac - b^2}
\end{aligned}
$$

Once the minimal distance points are obtained, the s_c and t_c are compared with the actual length of the cylinders in order to figure out which one should be kept as a cylinder, and which one should now be considered a disc. On Fig. 2.12 the bottom cylinder will be considered a disc, and the top one kept as a cylinder. As soon as this configuration is obtained, the calculation of the closest point between the two cylinders is straightforward: the center of the disc C_d is projected onto the line supporting the cylinder, and these two points define a vector V_{cl} which is re-projected onto the plane defined by the disc to get another vector $V_{discplane}$. Normalizing this vector and

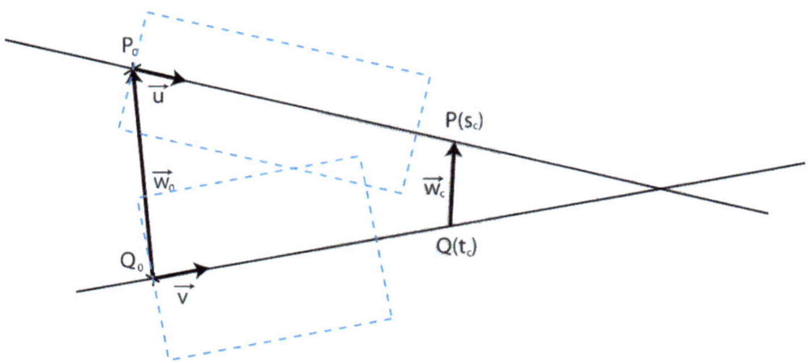

Fig. 2.12 Computation of the minimal distance between two lines. Each line is defined by a pair point-vector and the minimal distance points defining the unique vector which is perpendicular to both lines. In dashed lines are the two cylinders supported by the lines

multiply it by the radius of the disc gives us the closest point of the disc and from this closest point one can easily obtain the corresponding point of the cylinder.

Of course, this configuration is not always the one encountered when dealing with collision cylinders. However, reducing the problem to a cylinder/disc collision is always possible except when the closest point between the two lines supporting the cylinders actually lie on both cylinders.

Moreover, the cylinders are connected through a hierarchy of joints and their relative positions are strongly bound to their joints configuration. Thus, knowing whether two cylinders are colliding is equivalent with calculating the distance between two joints. If this distance is below a given threshold (namely the sum of the two cylinders radius) then the cylinders are penetrating each others. This approach is computationally cheaper than calculating the actual penetration thus it was used in place of the exact calculation for the optimization algorithms.

2.5.3 Arms Adaptation

The adaptation of the arms motion is done in two stages in order to reduce the computational complexity. First the penetration itself is removed, and then the motion is adapted so that it better matches the original.

2.5.3.1 Penetration Removal

This stage of the adaptation simply consists in rotating the shoulder joints so that the elbow remains at a threshold distance from the torso. Because there is only one joint being rotated, it exists an analytical solution. Considering in 2D the local reference frame depicted on Fig. 2.13, the target location for the elbow joint lies on the intersection of C_0 and C_1, the circles defined by the upper arm and threshold distance respectively. We pick a reference frame to make C_0 centered around the origin thus the equations of the two circles are: $x^2 + y^2 = l^2$ and $(x - x_j)^2 + (y - y_j)^2 = d^2$ respectively.

Developing these two equations gives yields to a second order equation on y, and re-injecting its solutions into the equation of C_0 gives the location of the target point for the elbow. The correction angle θ is then trivial to compute.

This 2D illustration can easily be extended to 3D by projecting the joints to the appropriate 2D plane.

This analytical solution gives one particular solution per frame, which might introduce discontinuities in the resulting motion. Thus we choose to use a global optimization approach instead. The goal here is to keep the elbow joint far away enough from the trunk so that no penetration remains. This is equivalent as keeping a minimal distance between two relevant joints, namely *elbow* and *spine*.

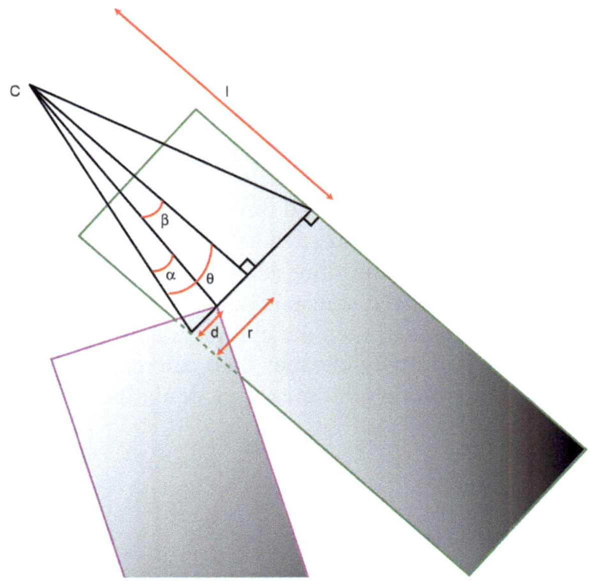

Fig. 2.13 Typical case of two cylinders penetrating each other. In green and violet are two cylinders. d is the penetration distance, l is the height between the center of rotation and the line supporting d, C the center of rotation of the joint that holds the green cylinder, α, β, θ are angles that must be calculated

Objective Function

We know in advance that the input motion exhibits some self penetration between the arms and the torso; otherwise it would be pointless to trigger the algorithm. Thus the starting point of the algorithm does not comply with the basic constraint we would like to enforce. It might turn out to be very difficult for the optimizer to find a good starting point. Moreover, we not only want to get a motion free of any self penetration, but we want also to change the joints angles as little as possible to keep the resulting motion as close as possible from the original. The objective function will thus be the sum of two functions, one for the penetration removal and one for the minimal corrections, as follows:

$$f(x) = \alpha x^2 + \beta \sum_m d_i(x) \quad x \in \mathbb{R}^n$$

$$d_i(x) = \begin{cases} \left(\left\| (P_i - Q_i) \right\| - d_{min} \right)^2 & \text{if} \left\| (P_i - Q_i) \right\| < d_{min} \\ 0 & \text{otherwise} \end{cases}$$

Here P_i and Q_i are the 3D position of the elbow and spine two joints at frame i and d_{min} is the minimal acceptable distance between the two joints. α and β are meant to make the optimizer first remove the penetrations and then minimize the corrections. In order to achieve so, the magnitude of the function related to the penetration should be at least one order of magnitude higher than the minimal corrections function. In our implementation, the correction angles were expressed in radians, while the distances were centimeters, and thus both α and β could be set to 1. x is a scalar representing the rotation of the shoulder joint. The rotation axis itself is dynamically chosen for each frame, so that the penetrations are removed with a minimal value of x.

2.5.3.2 Forearm Orientation Correction

The previous step made the motion of the arms self penetration free. However, its motion was changed and must be driven back towards its original configuration. What does being *close* from the original motion means? It all depends of what one wants to achieve. For instance, it could mean that the end effectors remain at their original location, for grasping objects for instance. As our focus was on catwalks, grasping something was not of great interest and instead we choose to bring back the forearm towards its initial orientation (Fig. 2.14).

There are still several degrees of freedom that remained untouched and it is over these ones that we will act. From the penetration removal, we know that two DoFs were used for this. Thus there is still one DoF of the shoulder and two more for the elbow which can be tweaked. At this stage, we will not use the elbow's DoF which makes the forearm rotate around itself because it does not help changing the forearm's orientation.

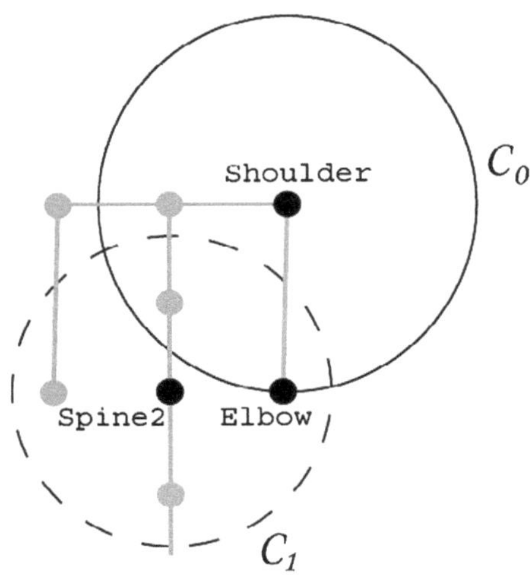

Fig. 2.14 Arms penetration removal. In grey is the skeleton and joints, in black the joints of interest, i.e. the shoulder, spine and elbow joints. Also in black the two circles used for the analytical calculation

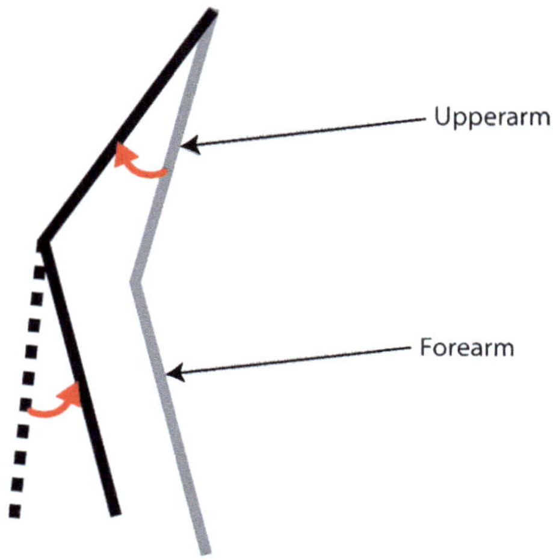

Fig. 2.15 Illustration of the arm adaptation process. In grey is the initial configuration of the arm. First the shoulder joint is rotated in order to drive the upper arm away from the body. The resulting configuration of the forearm has changed (*dashed lines*) and the elbow joint is thus rotated in order to bring the orientation of the forearm as close from the original one as possible

The objective function for this task is:

$$f(x) = -\sum_{m}(H_i - E_i)\cdot(h_i - e_i)$$

H_i and E_i are the original hand and elbow locations at frame i, while h_i and e_i are the new locations after the adaptation. No minimization of the correction is enforced this time, because we want the orientation to be as close from the original one as possible. Instead, to prevent the optimizer from adding big rotational values, constraints are added for all the available rotational DoFs, as follows (Fig. 2.15):

$$bg_j(x) = \begin{cases} -\dfrac{\pi}{2} - x_{\frac{j}{2}} & \text{if} \quad j \mod 2 = 0 \\ x_{\frac{j}{2}} - \dfrac{\pi}{2} & \text{otherwise} \end{cases}$$

The above set of constraints will bind the variables in two directions. This does not apply for the elbow rotation, as it only can be rotated in one direction. For this particular joint, the constraint functions thus become:

$$g_j(x) = \begin{cases} x_{\frac{j}{2}} & \text{if} \quad j \mod 2 = 0 \\ -x_{\frac{j}{2}} - \dfrac{\pi}{2} & \text{otherwise} \end{cases}$$

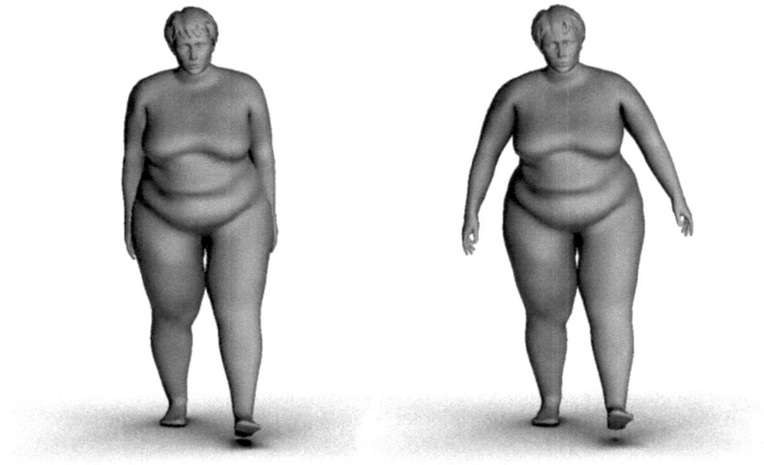

Fig. 2.16 Example of a penetration removal. On the right is the original posture, with the arms penetrating the body while on the right the arms are penetration free. The balance was also corrected on this example, however because the model was prepared by a designer beforehand the changes remained small

An example of such penetration removal can be seen on Fig. 2.16.

2.5.4 Legs Adaptation

The same way as the arms can self penetrate the body; the legs might have grown big enough to interpenetrate each other. The penetration might take place on the thigh or calf but this does not have a big impact on the algorithm we propose to address this issue. Again, for usual walking animations, detecting collisions between the two legs is equivalent with keeping a minimal distance between the calf joints. This is not true for more complex motions, e.g. if the character brings his foot towards his thigh, but we believe that in this case, a per-frame IK solution might be more adapted.

Getting rid of the self penetration in the case of walking does not allow for much freedom. Only the thigh joints can be touched straightforwardly, and the plump people often help themselves out by rotating their hip more than usual (Fig. 2.17). indeed, for a given posture and if the legs orientation is preserved, then rotating the hip helps to take the legs apart from each other. Thus, three DoFs (left thigh, right thigh and hip) are available for taking care of this penetration and among these three only two will be kept (the same correction values should be applied to both legs).

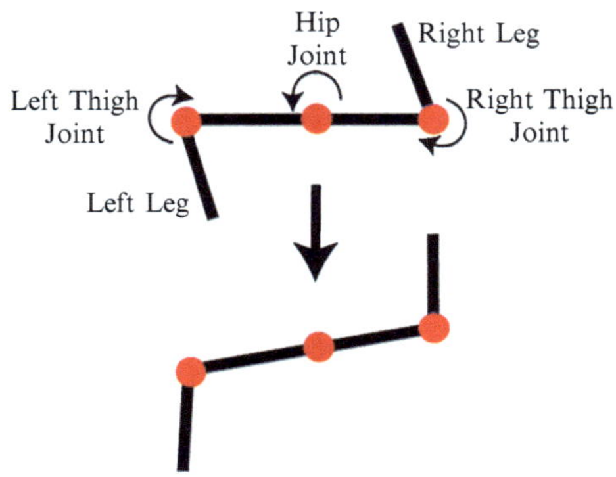

Fig. 2.17 Conceptual view of the legs configuration adaptation. The modifications are applied to the hip, left thigh and right thigh joints in order to drive the legs away from the body

The objective function associated with the legs resembles very much the one used for the arms penetration removal, as so:

$$f(x,y) = (\alpha x)^2 + (\beta y)^2 + \gamma \sum_m d_i(x,y) \quad x, y \in \mathbb{R}^n$$

$$d_i(x,y) \begin{cases} \left(\| (L_i - R_i) \| - d_{min} \right)^2 & \text{if} \, \| (L_i - R_i) \| < d_{min} \\ 0 & \text{otherwise} \end{cases}$$

This time, x represents the values of the hip rotation control points and y the thigh rotations, L_i and R_i are the left and right knee position at frame i (Fig. 2.17).

The squared distance used for the optimization works quite alright, but it fails to efficiently discriminate cases where the self collision might appear in the upper legs region, in the case of a very fat person for instance. This can be addressed by replacing the distance function of the previous equation by the following:

$$d_i(x,y) = \begin{cases} \left(\| M(L_i - R_i) \| - d_{min} \right)^2 & \text{if} \, \| M(L_i - R_i) \| < d_{min} \\ 0 & \text{otherwise} \end{cases}$$

Here M is a projection matrix that will project the points considered onto the plane defined by the vertical axis and the line between the left and right thigh joints. Conceptually, this has the effect of taking into account the actual separation of the legs, regardless of their configuration would they be close by (while standing for instance) or rather far apart (while walking).

A penetration might be removed by increasing the x or y values separately, thus the ratio between α and β determines whether it is the hip or thigh rotations that will take care of the issue. During our experiments, we noticed that a ratio of about 10 (i.e. $\beta = 10\alpha$) produces results which look quite natural.

2.5.5 General Purpose Collisions Removal

The arms and legs adaptation removed the penetrations related to the character shape. The remaining penetrations occur during a shorter amount of time, when the character puts its hand on its waist for instance. It is thus possible to use existing IK approaches to correct this. However, as we have the optimizer available to us, we propose to reuse it for this purpose. The principle remains the same, i.e. modify a given set of DoF so that no more penetration remains. The objective function becomes:

$$f(x) = (\alpha x)^2 + \beta \sum_J p_{ij} r_j^2 - d_{ij}^2$$

$$p_{ij} = \begin{cases} r_j^2 - d_{ij}^2 & \text{if } r_j^2 - d_{ij}^2 > 0 \\ 0 & \text{otherwise} \end{cases}$$

With x gathering the corrections of the DoF chosen for the adaptation, J the set of cylinders taken into account, r_j the radius of the jth cylinder and d_{ij} the distance at frame i between the colliding joint and the line supporting cylinder j. Better than a joint, it is straightforward to define one or several vertices of the body mesh that should not penetrate the body. Each vertex becomes an offset from its master joint, thus preventing a full deformation of the skin to calculate the value of f.

We implemented this algorithm and took into account the legs/torso, hands/torso, hands/head, hands/shoulder and hands/legs penetrations. We allowed the character to bend its elbow, rotate its shoulder and bend its torso depending on the kind of penetration considered. We placed control points every two frames because these collisions can occur within a short time.

2.5.6 Balance Correction

After the arms and legs penetration removal, the motion of the character has slightly changed and its balance is not maintained any longer. One last step takes place, so that the character's movement complies with the physical laws of motion.

The ZMP is of great importance to assess the balance of an animated figure. Its definition somewhat differs from publication to publication, but here is a way to think about it. When an avatar moves, the movements of its body creates momentum which yields to a force f and angular momentum m applied to the foot (or feet) in contact with the ground. f and m must be compensated for, otherwise the avatar collapses. f and m can be split into their horizontal and vertical components. The horizontal components of the force and vertical momentum can be accounted for by friction, as long as the foot remains in contact with the floor. The remaining components, however, must be compensated by the force generated by the ground reaction. Thus, the point where this force is exerted has to lie within the supporting polygon, otherwise the avatar cannot stop the ongoing motion. An extensive definition and discussion of the ZMP concept can be found in (Vukobratovic and Borovac 2004).

An active human body is rarely in equilibrium (Hudson 1996), and thus it often happens that this point goes out of the supporting polygon. Such a configuration does not mean that the person will necessarily fall, but rather that he/she must move his/her feet somewhere else before he/she collapses to the ground. For instance, during a normal walk cycle, the ZMP often goes out of the supporting area for a short instant. If something prevents the person from placing his/her other foot in front of him/her (step on the shoelace for instance), then he/she would actually fall straight to the floor. Oppositely, if the ZMP is inside the supporting area, this means that he/she has the ability to move towards an equilibrium state without having to reconfigure his/her foot plants. Because the momentum cannot be compensated for when it is outside of the supporting area, this point is often referred to as the Fictitious ZMP (FZMP).

2.5.6.1 Character Setup

Before to be able to act on the character's physical properties, the weights of the individual limbs must be estimated, along with the duration of the balanced and unbalanced states. This preprocessing is explained in the two following sections.

Weights Estimation

In order to perform an accurate adaptation of the character's gait, the weights of each of the character's limb must be known. In the case of a captured motion, the total weight of the subject being captured can be acquired at the same time, but even then this is not quite the data we are looking for. Moreover, assuming that the character's muscles can exert an arbitrary force, then the balance of a character is only bound by the distribution of its mass over its body and not by its total mass.

Thus the individual masses of the character's limb must be estimated. It is very difficult, if not impossible, to accurately measure the masses directly on the subject being captured. Because this issue arises as soon as one tries to deal with the physical properties of a movement, several studies were conducted in the past in order to get a meaningful estimate of the limb's density. For instance, the US army conducted series of measures on corpses (Chandler et al. 1975; Dempster 1955) and eventually came up with the density measures and masses percentages reproduced on the tables below.

Using this table and assuming that a particular limb's volume is known, it becomes straightforward to calculate the limb's mass. Previous work used global optimization in order to estimate these masses (Popovic and Witkin 1999). They calculate the optimal mass distribution so that the original motion clip would appear to be balanced throughout a given animation clip. However, we noticed that

Table 2.1 Mean density of body parts (Chandler et al. 1975)

Body part	Density (g/mm)
Head	1.056
Torso	0.853
Right upperarm	0.997
Left upperarm	1.012
Upperarms mean	1.0045
Right forearm	1.043
Left forearm	1.061
Forearms mean	1.052
Right hand	1.079
Left hand	1.081
Hands mean	1.080
Right thigh	1.018
Left thigh	1.021
Thighs mean	1.0195
Right calf	1.059
Left calf	1.079
Calf mean	1.069
Right foot	1.073
Left foot	1.073
Feet mean	1.071

this optimization easily fails to accurately estimate the masses, but often falls into local minima with an unrealistic mass distribution. Instead we decided to calculate this data from the limb's volume along with the densities from Table 2.1.

Another way to proceed would have been to calculate the entire volume of the body using for instance the method proposed by Muller (Müller et al. 2007) and to use Table 2.2 to allocate a specific percentage of the total mass to each limb. Again, the actual total mass of the character is of little interest here because the balance is not modified by a global weight scale.

For the limbs' volume calculation, we relied on a cylindrical model of the body (Hanavan and Ernest 1964) because it also provides the center of mass associated with each limb. This enables to directly calculate the ZMP of the character from a given animated clip.

Threshold Distances Calculation

During dynamically balanced motion, it is commonly admitted in the CG community that the ZMP should remain within the supporting area of the character. This, to our experience (c.f. Section 2.5.6) is not always the case. Thus, instead of bringing the ZMP back within this polygon, we calculate it for the original motion and body shape. This gives one distance zmpi between the ZMP and supporting area for each frame i, distance which is used as a per-frame threshold during the balance correction (Fig. 2.18).

Table 2.2 Percentage of the body parts compared to the entire body (Dempster 1955)

Body part	Percentage of the total body mass (%)
Trunk minus limbs	56.5
Trunk minus limbs and shoulders	46.9
Shoulders	10.3
Head and neck	7.9
Thorax	11.0
Abdomen and pelvis	26.4
Entire upper left extremity	4.8
Left upperarm	2.6
Left forearm and hand	2.1
Left forearm	1.5
Left hand	0.6
Entire upper right extremity	4.9
Right upperarm	2.7
Right forearm and hand	2.2
Right forearm	1.6
Right hand	0.6
Entire lower left extremity	15.7
Left thigh	9.7
Left leg and foot	6.0
Left leg	4.5
Left foot	1.4
Entire lower right extremity	15.7
Right thigh	9.6
Right leg and foot	5.9
Right leg	4.5
Right foot	1.4

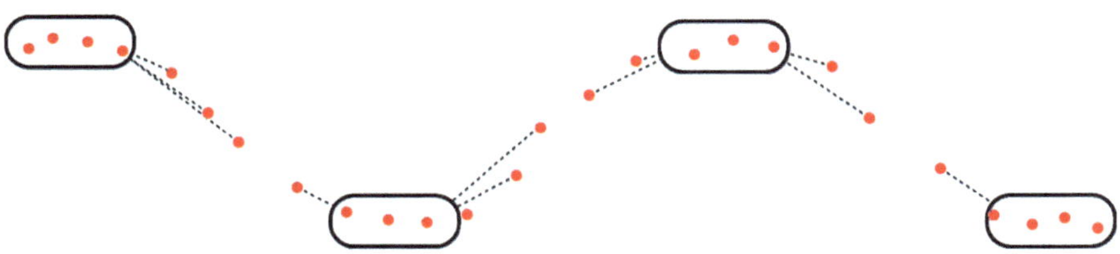

Fig. 2.18 Illustration of the balanced frame concept. In black are four successive supporting areas, and in red are several calculated ZMPs. The dashed lines are the threshold distance zmpi that are kept for each frame of the animation

2.5.6.2 Balance Optimization

The ZMP is given by the following formula, which defines the point where the total torque due to both body acceleration and gravity is null:

$$\sum_i (r_i - Z) \times (m_i(\ddot{r}_i - g)) = 0$$

with r_i the location of the center of mass of body i, ri its acceleration, mi its mass, Z the ZMP and g the gravity acceleration. A direct calculation of Z is possible through (Tak and Ko 2005):

$$ZMP = \begin{pmatrix} \dfrac{\sum_i m_i(\ddot{y}_i + g)x_i - \sum_i m_i \ddot{x}_i y_i}{\sum_i m_i(\ddot{y}_i + g)} \\ \dfrac{\sum_i m_i(\ddot{y}_i + g)z_i - \sum_i m_i \ddot{z}_i y_i}{\sum_i m_i(\ddot{y}_i + g)} \end{pmatrix} i \varepsilon R$$

with R the set of rigid bodies composing the character, and m_i is the mass associated with rigid body i. Due to the second derivative terms, this calculation involves several consecutive frames, thus a per-frame approach is not applicable here.

The goal here is to bring back the ZMP closer than zmp_i from the supporting area (Fig. 2.19). For doing so, we move the Center of Mass (CoM) of the character using the ankle and thigh articulations or lean the torso (Fig. 2.20). We allow the optimization to use both these strategies by defining four free sets of variables: two for the legs adaptation and two for the torso. Each pair of variables makes the CoM move sideways or forward/backward.

The torso variables can directly be applied to the spine joint of the character, while the legs variables are shared by the ankle and thigh joints with the appropriate sign value. Because a distance from a supporting area is analog to a penetration, we can reuse the same optimization strategy. Here the objective function for the balance becomes:

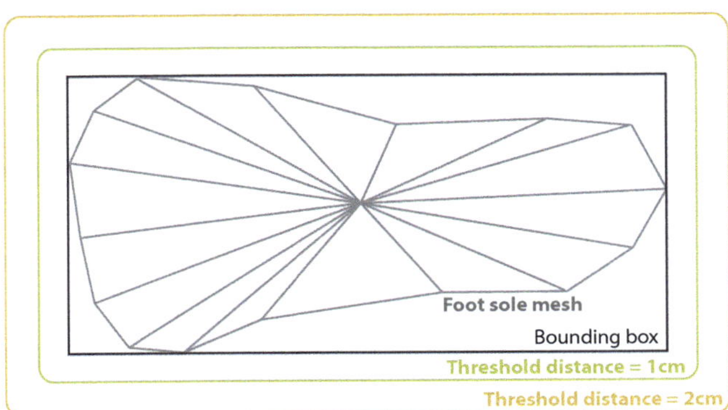

Fig. 2.19 Illustration of the supporting area and threshold distances calculation. In grey is the foot sole mesh. First its bounding box is extracted so that it can be used as supporting area. From this bounding box, the acceptable area for the ZMP is calculated. The area depends on the maximal acceptable distance between the ZMP and the supporting area, as seen with the two example areas (in *green* and *orange*)

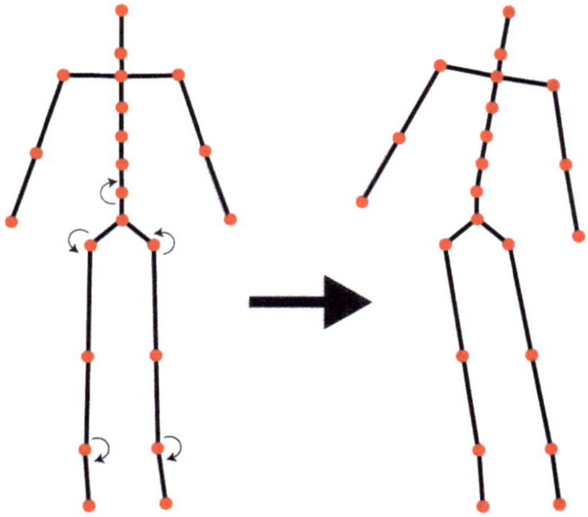

Fig. 2.20 Conceptual view of the balance adaptation. The legs move the CoM towards the left, while the torso is bent so that the CoM moves in the opposite direction

$$f(x) = \alpha \|x\|_1 + \beta \sum_x d_i(x) \quad x \in \mathbb{R}^n$$

$$d_{i(x)} = \begin{cases} \|(S_i - \mathrm{ZMP}_i)\| - d_{\max} & \text{if } \|(S_i - \mathrm{ZMP})\| > d_{\max} \\ 0 & \textit{otherwise} \end{cases}$$

Here $\alpha = 10$ and $\beta = 1$. ZMP_i is the location of the ZMP at frame i, S_i is the closest point from the ZMP on the supporting area and d_{max} is the maximal distance from the supporting area allowed for the ZMP.

As for the arms constraints, some local minimum of $f(x)$ might be achieved by non realistic (and impossible) configurations of the limbs. Hence we also impose bounds on the values of x, i.e. the corrections applied to the motion cannot exceed a given value, as follows:

$$g_j(x) = \begin{cases} x_{\frac{j}{2}} - \frac{\pi}{8} & \text{if } j \bmod 2 = 0 \\ -x_{\frac{j}{2}} - \frac{\pi}{8} & \text{otherwise} \end{cases}$$

Examples of such adaptation can be seen on Figs. 2.21–2.23.

2.5.6.3 Runtime System

As explained in the previous sections, modifying the character's motion takes quite some time due to the several non-linear optimizations that take place during the

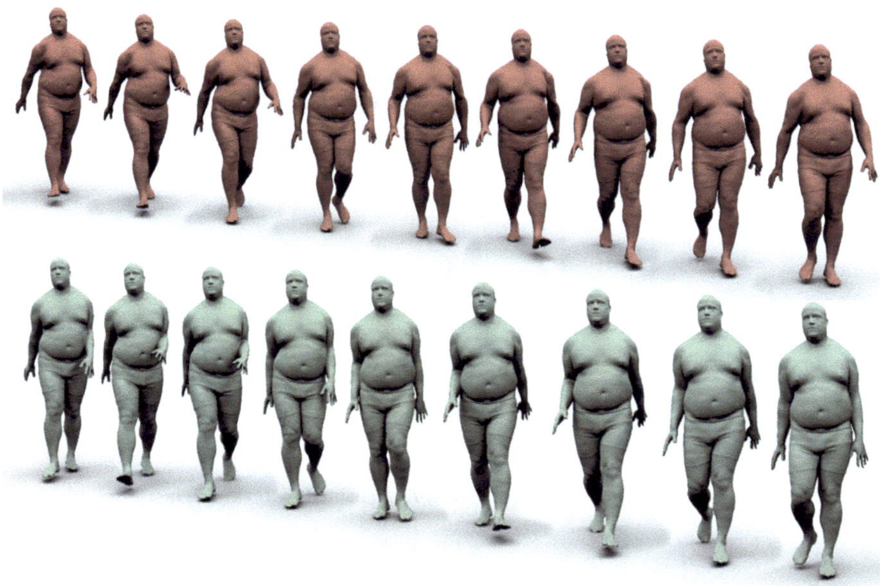

Fig. 2.21 Walking character. *Top*: adapted, *bottom*: original

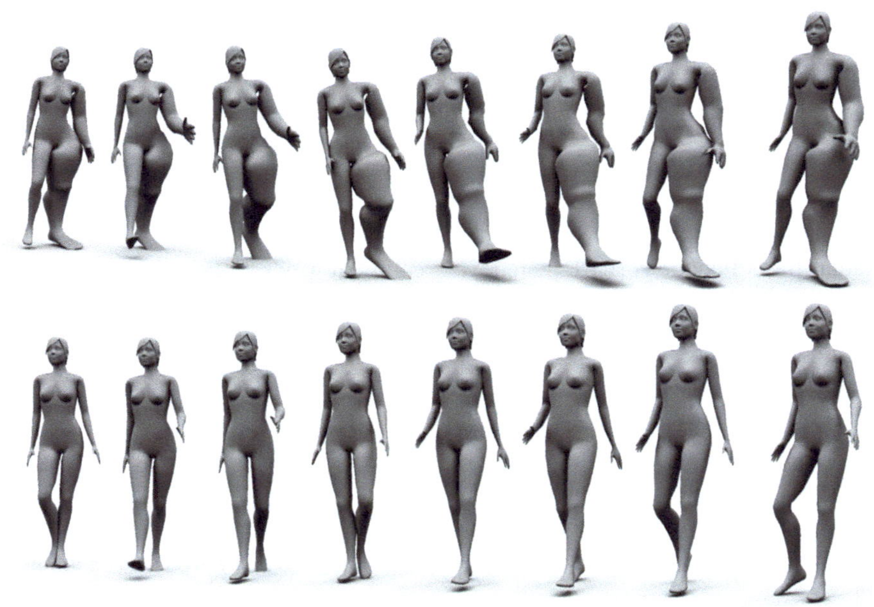

Fig. 2.22 Grown character: the original mesh was deformed to larger its leg. *Top*: grown and adapted, *bottom*: original

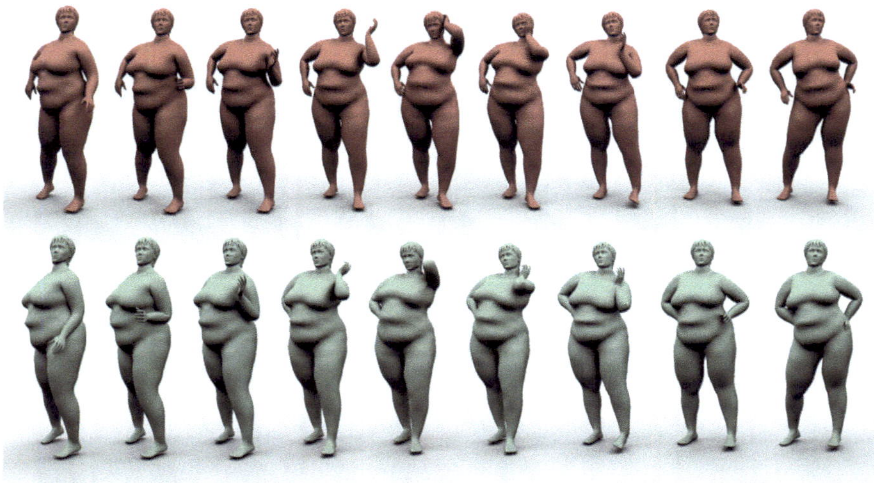

Fig. 2.23 A character posing with self-collisions. *Top*: adapted, *bottom*: original

process. Thus, in view of the use within a VTO application, the adaptation related to a specific character's sizes should be achieve at least in interactive time. In order to overcome this issue, we devised a framework that pre-calculates the corrections for a given number of examples shapes, and interpolates these at run time in order to quickly come up with adequate corrections. To do so, we use scattered data interpolation techniques, which have proven to be efficient for this purpose.

Radial Basis Functions

Radial Basis Functions (RBFs) are a very common way to interpolate an example data set in order to estimate the value of intermediate samples. The most common formulation of a RBF $\varphi : \Re^n \rightarrow \Re$ is:

$$\varphi(X) = \sum_{i=1}^{N} a_i \rho\left(\|X - C_i\|\right)$$

with N the number example data points, C_i the center vector of example data i, a_i is the weight associate with the example data i and ρ an interpolating function.

A better formulation, called normalized radial basis function (NRBF) is as follows:

$$\varphi(X) = \frac{\sum_{i=1}^{N} a_i \rho\left(\|X - C_i\|\right)}{\sum_{i=1}^{N} \rho\left(\|X - C_i\|\right)}$$

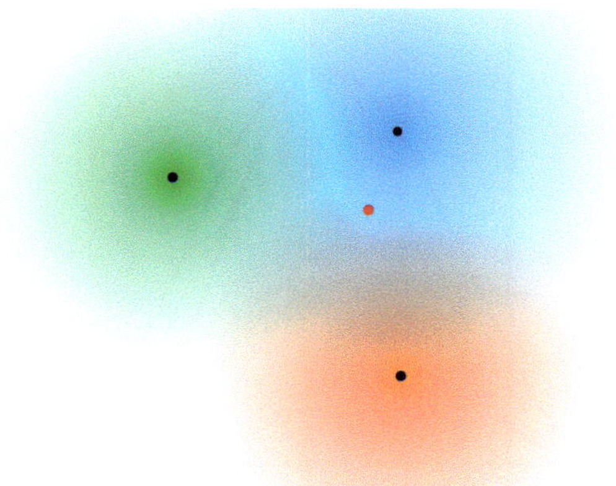

Fig. 2.24 Conceptual principle of a radial basis function. Here in this 2D example, three sample data points (*black dots*) each have an influence over their neighboring regions (*colored area*), and a new point (*red dot*) can be interpolated by taking into account the influence and confidence of the example data

A theoretical justification of this formulation can be found in (Buhmann and Ablowitz 2003). Intuitively, RBFs simply are a way to calculate a data sample by a weighted interpolation of existing data (Fig. 2.24) If the sum of the interpolated data is not equal to 1, then the resulting data will not properly reflect the examples and should thus be normalized, hence the normalized formulation.

The most commonly chosen function for ρ is to use a Gaussian:

$$\rho(x) = \exp[-\beta x^2]$$

Gaussians are considered local in the sense that their value decreases to 0 when tending towards infinity. In our case, we have the possibility to choose where the example data point will be taken in the data space. If we choose an adequate function for ρ, then it is possible to accurately re-synthesize the existing data points. By adequate we mean that the function should truly be local and not just only tend towards 0. Moreover, it should have the nice interpolation properties of the Gaussian function so that the interpolation remains smooth.

The hanning function (Press et al. 1992) is commonly used in signal processing (Blackman and Tukey 1959) and appears to have all the desired properties:

$$h(t) = \begin{cases} 0.5 - 0.5\cos\left(2\pi \dfrac{t}{T}\right) & t \in [0,T] \\ 0 \text{ otherwise} \end{cases}$$

Its value really is 0 outside the defined bounds, and its shape is almost the same as the Gaussian within the interpolation range (Fig. 2.25). By using this function in

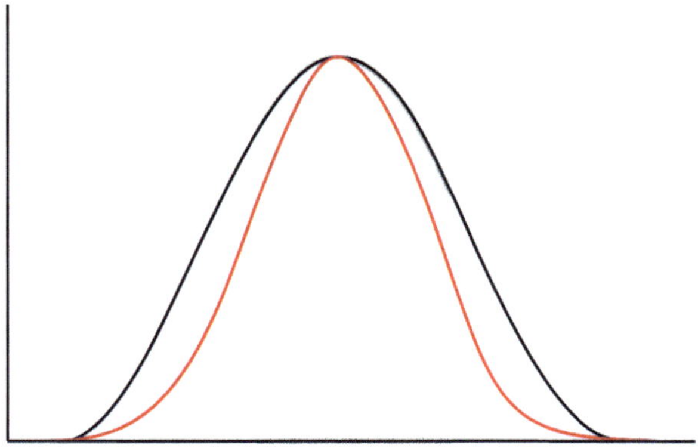

Fig. 2.25 Comparison between gauss (in *red*) and hanning (in *black*) functions. The functions parameters were chosen so that the center and span of each function matches

place of a Gaussian, we can truly limit the influence of the sample through the interpolation space.

Regarding the distance function, the Euclidian distance is the most commonly used one. However, its equidistant lines are circular and thus the influence of a particular example point cannot strictly be bound between square areas. Instead, we use the infinity norm (also known as Chebyshev distance) defined as follows:

$$d_{Cheb}(p,q) = \lim_{k \to \infty} \left(\sum_{i=1}^{N} |p_i - q_i|^k \right)^{1/K}$$

With p and q n-dimensional vectors.

Fortunately, it is easy to calculate this infinite norm: $d_{Cheb}(p,q) = \max_i(|p_i - q_i|)$. This distance corresponds much better to our needs because equidistant lines draw hypercubes in the computation space instead of hyperspheres (Fig. 2.26). Thus if the example data samples are regularly spaced in all the interpolation dimensions, we can smoothly interpolate between the samples and guarantee that the calculated data points accurately reflect the example data set.

Data Pre-processing

A customizable body model is usually composed of about 30 segments which can be individually deformed. Even though the arms and legs adaptation only rely on the size of the arms and legs, the balance correction is dependent on the individual growth of each of the segments. Thus, in order to take into account all of the subtle equilibrium change induced by each of the body segments, we would have to make each segment vary individually to cover the entire interpolation space. In that case, the interpolation space would have 30 dimensions and if we want to calculate three states for each variable (small, neutral and big) then the number of optimizations to

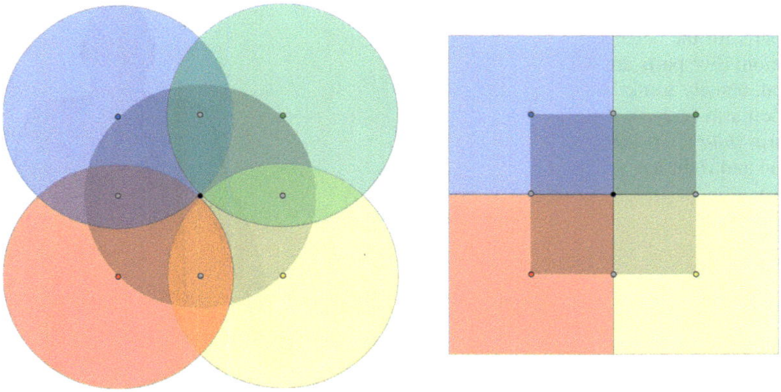

Fig. 2.26 Comparison between the use of the Euclidian distance (*left*) and the infinity norm (*right*) in 2D. On the left, equidistant lines draw spheres while the infinity norm draws squares. If the sample data points are regularly spaced, this enables to accurately re-synthesize and interpolate the sample data set

perform would be 3^{30}, obviously a number way too big to be tractable in practice. Instead, we reduced the number of variables to five, namely the size of both legs, the trunk and both arms (Fig. 2.27). This simplification still yields to good results in practice because the variation of individual segments within a particular limb only little influence the final result as long and the global modification of the limb is taken into account.

Each limb is successively reduced and grown in diameter while keeping the other limbs size fixed. The number of optimizations to perform is thus $3^5 = 243$ which takes approximately 10 h on a Pentium 4 3.0 GHz for a 800 frames animation. The pre-calculated example data can then be interpolated by NRBF with the hanning function and Chebyshev distance.

Skeleton Adaptation

Adapting the motion of a character is meant to make its animation more suited to its actual shape. When an arbitrary character and animation are given to the system, there is no way to know whether the animation was already prepared by a designer or not. Hence, it is quite reasonable to assume that the skeleton provided with the body should not be modified. In the case of a deformable body, the character shape and skeleton are provided in neutral configuration and can be modified in order to make it smaller or bigger. As we know what the skeletal configuration for the standard shape is, it is possible to modify the associated skeleton so that it better match the shape before performing the motion adaptation, as explained in the following section.

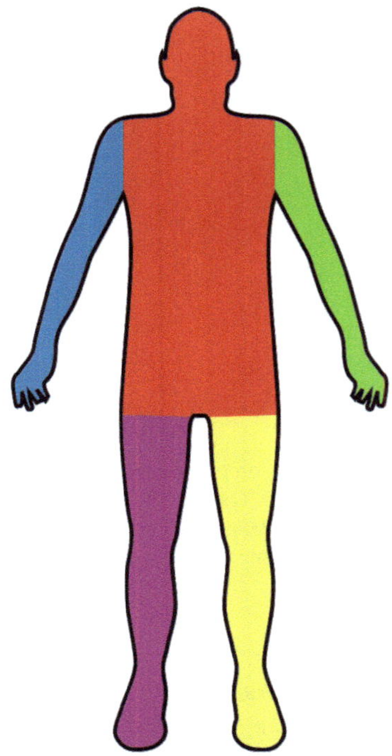

Fig. 2.27 Split of the body parts for the balance correction. Five parts are retained, namely trunk (*red*), left arm (*green*), right arm (*blue*), left leg (*yellow*) and right leg (*purple*)

A Growing Body

It exists several ways to accurately deform a body shape so that it has specific dimensions. Seo (Seo and Magnenat-Thalmann 2003) proposed a method based on examples which are later interpolated with RBFs to produce new shapes with the desired features. This example based approach has one important drawback in the sense that because only examples are interpolated (mostly shapes from 3D scanners) then the resulting shapes resemble very much the input data and thus will exhibit very realistic but somewhat ugly features of the human body. Allen (Allen et al. 2003) proposed a parametric approach to achieve the same goal. The way a body is deformed is defined by the user and can thus be very well bound to aesthetic shapes.

Both approaches require a fair amount of manual work in order to obtain visually pleasing shapes. Instead of using either one of these two we decided to propose a much simpler approach which even though it does not produce very pretty shapes is fast to implement and to use. Moreover, because we used this approach only for testing our motion adaptation algorithms, we did not care so much about the visual aspect of the resulting bodies.

Our method relies on the skin attachment on the body along with the skeleton design in order to estimate how each vertex should be moved. To understand what the skin attachment means, one should know how the skin is deformed. We implemented the linear blend skinning method proposed by Magnenat-Thalmann et al. (1988). Even though quite simple, this approach is still widely used for interactive applications and can be expressed as follows:

$$v_i' = \sum_j M_j B_j^{-1} v_i$$

with M_j the current transformation matrix of joint j, B_j the bind transform matrix of joint j, v_i the initial position of vertex i in bind pose, v_i' the deformed location of vertex i.

Conceptually, each vertex is attached to one or more joints, with a weight associated to each influencing joint. The sum of the weights is equal to 1, and they are carefully chosen so that the character smoothly deforms along with the skeleton motion. In order to be computationally efficient, the product $B_j^{-1} v_i$ from equation is pre computed for each vertex, and thus each vertex is stored as a collection of offsets from their respective influencing bones, in local coordinates.

Additionally, the skeleton is done in such a way that the x axis of the bones are oriented towards the next joint. Considering that the limbs length do not change, then the growth of a limb is done by scaling the offsets in the y and z directions, as follows:

$$W_i = \Sigma_j w_j$$

$$W'_i = \frac{\Sigma_k W_k}{K} k \in K$$

$$\begin{cases} o_{ix} = o_{ix} \\ o_{iy} = o_{iy} + (\alpha - 1) \cdot o_{iy} \cdot W'_i \\ o_{iz} = o_{iz} + (\alpha - 1) \cdot o_{iz} \cdot W'_i \end{cases}$$

with w_j the weight associated to the jth influencing bone of vertex i, K the set of vertices directly connected to vertex i, α the scaling factor and o_i the offsets of vertex i. An example of such growth can be seen on Fig. 2.28.

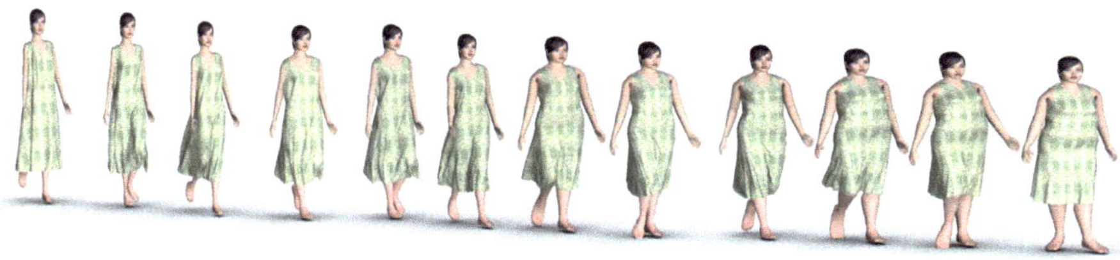

Fig. 2.28 Snapshots of a walking sequence of a deformable character growing along its path. The adaptation data was pre-calculated and interpolated at runtime to adapt the animation according to the character's growth. A foot skating removal algorithm was applied afterward in order to get rid of the induced foot skating

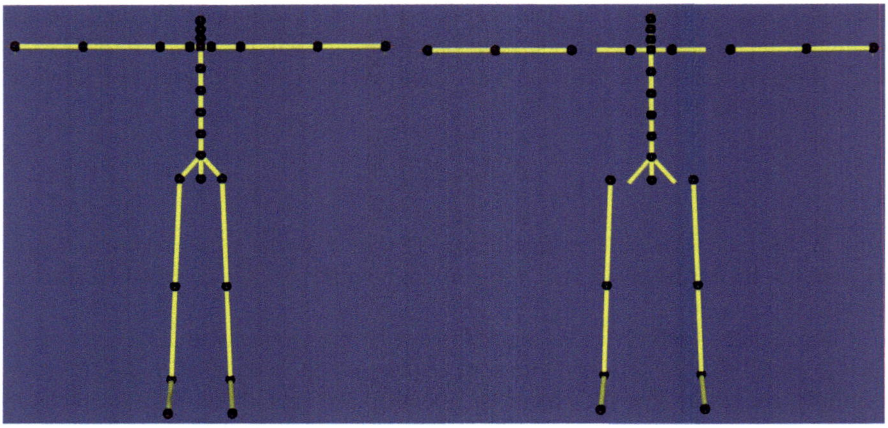

Fig. 2.29 Scaling of the skeleton segments according to the growth imposed on the offsets. On the left is the original skeleton, while on the right is the scaled skeleton after a growth by a factor of 2.0. Note the gap at the clavicle and thigh joints

Joints Translation

When the body grows, its joints should be resized accordingly. It is straightforward to estimate the scale that must be applied when the length of a segment is changed; however changing the girth of the trunk may also induce a skeleton resizing. Figure 2.10 shows that six segments connect the spine to the limbs, namely the clavicle, upper arm and thigh segments. Thus, when scaling the trunk by a factor α, these segments will also be scaled by the same factor, as seen on Fig. 2.29. Depending on the magnitude of the scale, it might be possible to deal with the changes by only adapting the motion. However, we noticed that we obtain much better results by also taking into account the resizing of the skeleton.

References

Abe Y., Liu K., Popovic Z.: Momentum-based parameterization of dynamic character motion. Graph. Models, 68(2):194–211, Academic Press Professional, Inc. (2006)

Allen B., Curless B., Popovic Z.: The space of human body shapes: reconstruction and parameterization from range scans. SIGGRAPH '03: ACM SIGGRAPH 2003 Papers, 587–594, (2003)

Baerlocher P., Boulic R.: An inverse kinematic architecture enforcing an arbitrary number of strict priority levels. The Visual Computer, 20(6):402–417, Springer-Verlag, New York, (2003)

Betts J.T., Smith R.: Practical methods for optimal control using nonlinear programming. Society for Industrial and Applied Mathematics, Philadelphia, PA, (2001)

Bindiganavale R., Badler N.I.: Motion abstraction and mapping with spatial contraints. In CAPTECH '98: Proceedings of the international workshop on modelling and motion capture techniques for virtual environments, 70–82, London, UK, Springer-Verlag, (1998)

Blackman R.B., Tukey J.W.: The measurement of power spectra, from the point of view of communications Engineering. Dover Plublications, (1959)
Boulic R., Huang Z., Thalmann D.: A comparison of design strategies for 3D human motions. In human comfort and security of information systems; Advanced interface for the Information Society, 19–21, Springer-Verlag, (1997)
Boulic R., Le Callennec B., Herren M., Bay H.: Experimenting prioritized ik for motion editing. In: Proceedings of Eurographics, (2003)
Bruderlin A., Williams L.: Motion signal processing. In: Proceedings of the 22nd annual conference on computer graphics and interactive techniques, 97–104, (1995)
Buhmann M.D., Ablowitz M.J.: Radial basis functions: theory and implementations. Cambridge University Press, (2003)
Catmull E., Rom R.: A class of local interpolating splines. Computer aided geometric design, 317–326 (1974)
Chai J., Hodgins J.K.: Constraint-based motion optimization using a statistical dynamic model. In: SIGGRAPH '07: ACM SIGGRAPH 2007 Papers, p. 8, New York, (2007)
Chandler R.F., Clauser C.E., McConville J.T., Reynolds H.M., Young J.W.: Investigation of intertial properties of the human body. US Department of Transportation report, (1975)
Choi K.J., Ko H.S.: Online motion retargeting. Journal of Visualization and Computer Animation, 11(5):223–235, (2000)
Cohen M.F.: Interactive spacetime control for animation. SIGGRAPH Comput Graph, 26(2):293–302, (1992)
Dempster W.T.: Space requirements of the seated operator. Wright Air Development Center report-55-159, (1955)
Glardon P., Boulic R., Thalmann D.: Robust on-line adaptive footplant detection and enforcement for locomotion. Vis Comput 22(3):194–209, (2006)
Gleicher M.: Motion editing with spacetime constraints. In: Proceedings of SI3D'97 symposium on interactive 3D graphics, p. 139-ff, New York, ACM Press, (1997)
Gleicher M.: Retargeting motion to new characters. In: Proceedings of SIGGRAPH 1998, Computer graphics proceedings, Annual conference series, ACM Press/ACM SIGGRAPH, 33–42, (1998)
Hanavan J., Ernest P.: A mathematical model of the human body. USAF report, (1964)
Hudson J.L.: Biomechanics of balance: paradigms and procedures. Proceedings of the XIIIth international symposium on biomechanics in sports, 286–289, (1996)
Ikemoto L., Arikan O., Forsyth D.: Knowing when to put your foot down. I3D '06: Proceedings of the 2006 symposium on interactive 3D graphics and games, 49–53, New York, ACM Press, (2006)
Jeong K., Lee S.: Motion adaptation with self-intersection avoidance. In: Proceedings of the international workshop on human modeling and animation, 77–85, (2000)
Kovar L., Schreiner J., Gleicher M.: Footskate cleanup for motion capture editing. Proceedings of the ACM symposium on computer animation, 97–104, New York, ACM Press, (2002)
Kuffner J., Nishiwaki K., Kagami S., Kuniyoshi Y., Inaba M., Inoue H.: Self-collision detection and prevention for humanoid robots. In international conference on robotics and automation, 2265–2270, IEEE, (2002)
Lee J., Shin S.Y.: A hierarchical approach to interactive motion editing for human-like figures. In: Proceedings of SIGGRAPH 1999, Computer graphics proceedings, Annual conference series, 39–48, ACM, ACM Press/ACM SIGGRAPH, New York, (1999)
Liu K.C., Hertzmann A., Popovic Z.: Composition of complex optimal multi-character motions. SCA '06: Proceedings of the 2006 ACM SIGGRAPH/Eurographics symposium on computer animation, 215–222, (2006)
Magnenat-Thalmann N., Laperrière R., Thalmann D.: Joint-dependent local deformations for hand animation and object grasping. Proceedings on graphics interface '88, 26–33, Toronto, ON, (1988)
Müller M., Heidelberger B., Hennix M., Ratcliff J.: Position based dynamics. J Vis Cmun Image Represent, 18(2):109–118, (2007)

Nickalls R.W.D.: A new approach to solving the cubic: cardan's solution revealed. Math Gazette, 77:354–359, (1993)
Peinado M., Boulic R., Le Callennec B., Meziat D.: Progressive cartesian inequality constraints for the inverse kinematics control of articulated chains. In Eurographics, short presentation session, 93–96, Eurographics Association, (2005)
Peinado M., Meziat D., Raunhardt D., Boulic R.: Environment-aware postural control of virtual humans for real-time applications. In of the SAE conference on digital human modeling for design and engineering, (2006)
Peinado M., Meziat D., Maupu D., Raunhardt D., Thalmann D., Boulic R.: Accurate on-line avatar control with collision anticipation. In VRST '07: Proceedings of the 2007 ACM symposium on virtual reality software and technology, 89–97, New York, ACM Press, (2007)
Ponder M., Papagiannakis G., Molet T., Magnenat-Thalmann N., Thalmann D.: VHD++ development framework: towards extendible, component based VR/AR simulation engine featuring advanced virtual character technologies, Proceedings of computer graphics international (CGI), IEEE Computer Society Press, (2003)
Popovic Z.: Controlling physics in realistic character animation. Commun ACM, 43(7):50–58, (2000)
Popovic Z., Witkin A.: Motion warping. In: Proceedings of SIGGRAPH 1995, Computer graphics proceedings, Annual conference series, New York, ACM, ACMPress/ACMSIGGRAPH, (1995)
Popovic Z., Witkin A.: Physically based motion transformation. In: Proceedings of SIGGRAPH 1999, Computer graphics proceedings, Annual conference series, 11–20, New York, ACM, ACM Press/ACM SIGGRAPH, (1999)
Press W.H., Flannery B.P., Tukolsky S.A., Vetterling W.T.: Numerical recipes in C: the art of scientific computing (2nd edn). Cambridge University Press, (1992)
Seo H., Magnenat-Thalmann N.: An automatic modeling of human bodies from sizing parameters. ACM SIGGRAPH 2003 symposium on interactive 3D graphics, 19–26, ACM Press, (2003)
Shin H.J., Kovar L., Gleicher M.: Physical touch-up of human motions. In: Proceedings of the pacific conference on computer graphics and applications, p. 194, IEEE Computer Society, Wiley-IEEE Computer Society Press, (2003)
Tak S., Ko H.S.: A physically-based motion retargeting filter. ACM Trans Graph, 24(1):98–117, (2005)
The VR Juggler-Open Source Virtual Reality Tools. http://www.vrjuggler.org/. Accessed April 2008 (2008)
Tolani D., Goswami A., Badler N.I.: Real-time inverse kinematics techniques for anthropomorphic limbs. Graph Model, 62:353–388, (2000)
Vukobratovic M., Borovac B.: Zero-moment point – thirty five years of its life. Int J Human Robot, 1(1):157–173, World Scientific Publishing, (2004)
Witkin A., Kass M.: Spacetime constraints. In: Proceedings of SIGGRAPH 1988, Computer graphics proceedings, Annual conference series. ACM, ACM Press/ACM SIGGRAPH, 159–168, New York, (1988)
Zhao X., Badler N.: Interactive body awareness. Comput-Aid Design, 26(12):861–866, Elsevier Science, (1994)

Chapter 3
Cloth Modeling and Simulation

Abstract This chapter addresses techniques for cloth modeling and simulation. After a brief introduction to the historic background of garment simulation in computer graphics, the chapter describes methods for measuring the physical parameters of textile materials. The core of the chapter is given by the section on the physical simulation of cloth. The addressed topics range from the generalities of mechanical simulation and state-of-the-art techniques to the description of a simple method for accurate simulation of nonlinear cloth materials, covering also numerical integration, collision handling and real-time animation issues. The chapter ends with a section on the haptic interaction with virtual textiles which describes the problems to solve when touching cloth-like deformable objects in a virtual reality environment and includes a case study detailing the research and development of a prototype interface designed for the haptic simulation of cloth.

3.1 A Brief History on Garment Simulation

Garment simulation, which has started in the late eighties with very simple models, has taken a tremendous benefit of the progressing computer hardware and tools as well as the development of specific simulation technologies which have nowadays lead to impressive applications not only in the field of simulation of virtual worlds, but also as design tools for the garment and fashion industry.

In the field of computer graphics, the first applications for cloth simulation appeared in 1987 (Terzopoulos et al. 1987) in the form of a simulation system relying on the Lagrange equations of motion and elastic surface energy. Solutions were obtained through finite difference schemes on regular grids. This allowed, for example, the accurate simulation of a flag or the draping of a rectangular cloth and could distinguish it from any stiff material such as a metal, or plastic.

Such a mechanical model was used to produce one of the first animated virtual garments, in the form of a skirt animated by blowing air in the sequence "Flashback" (Lafleur and Magnenat-Thalmann 1991). Through the very limited computational power at this time, only the moving skirt cone was simulated, and collisions were

N. Magnenat-Thalmann (ed.), *Modeling and Simulating Bodies and Garments*,
DOI 10.1007/978-1-84996-263-6_3,

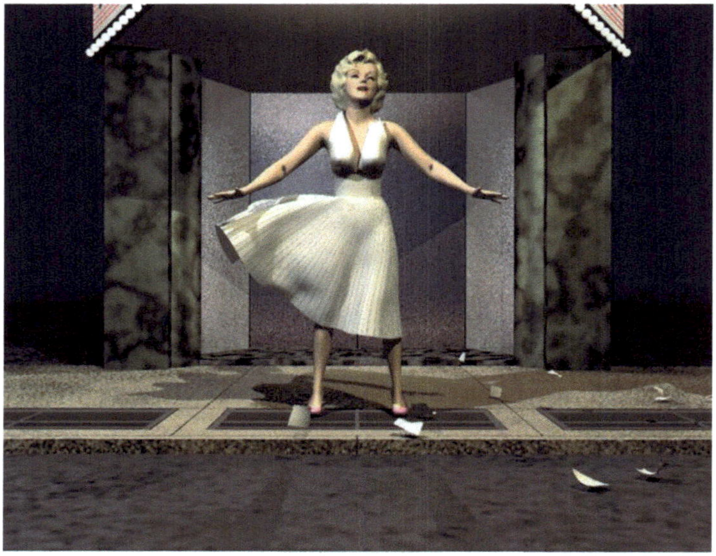

Fig. 3.1 "Flashback" (Lafleur and Magnenat-Thalmann 1991)

handled through simple repulsion forces over a simplified representation of the pelvis and legs (Fig. 3.1).

At the meantime, the development of other topics such as body modeling and animation and collision detection and response has led to the improvement of versatile garment simulation in more general contexts (Carignan and Magnenat-Thalmann 1992; Yang and Magnenat-Thalmann 1993), taking advantage of basic pattern-based design systems (Werner et al. 1993) (Fig. 3.2).

Since then, many new advances in the field of cloth simulation models have improved achievements in virtual garments. Among major developments, new particle-system approaches have led to specific cloth simulation systems more adapted to the large deformability of cloth and contact processing (Breen et al. 1994; Volino et al. 1995; Eberhardt et al. 1996). In parallel, collision detection techniques have also been improved, mostly through the use of hierarchical techniques taking advantage of some geometrical specificities of cloth surfaces and context-dependent optimizations, allowing the processing of much more complex garments, with multiple cloth layers and wrinkles handled through self-collision processing (Volino and Magnenat-Thalmann 1994). These developments have led to the possibility of simulating garments in much wider contexts than simply being worn by a character (Fig 3.3).

Through the use of these techniques, garment simulation improved in maturity, and advanced design options became available (Volino et al. 1997), bringing some new possibilities of creating or duplicating actual fashion models (Fig. 3.4).

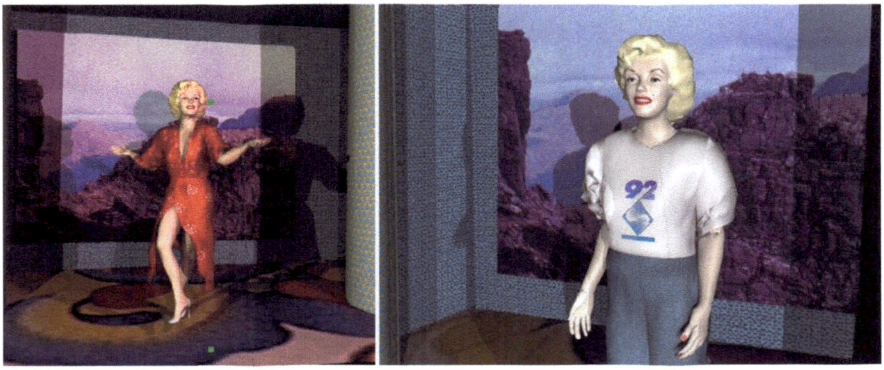

Fig. 3.2 "Fashion Show", early models of dressed virtual characters (Carignan and Magnenat-Thalmann 1992)

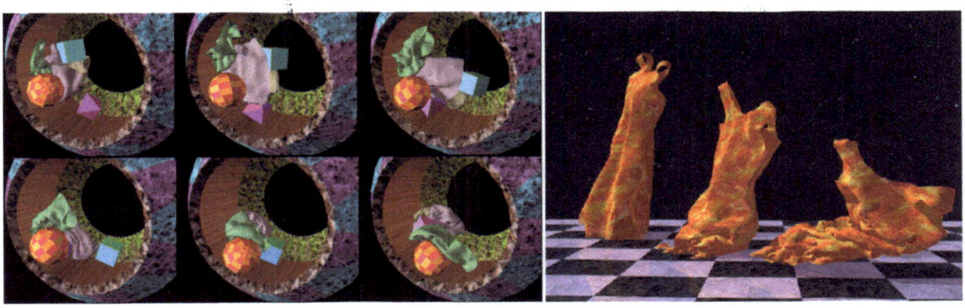

Fig. 3.3 General garment simulation using advanced collision processing techniques (Volino et al. 1995)

While the results obtained through these techniques were acceptable for computer graphics purposes, whey were still not sufficiently accurate to fulfill the requirements of CAD and Virtual Prototyping applications required by the garment industry.

For fulfilling these new goals, cloth simulation techniques required some improvements and maturations, which first came through the use of implicit numerical integration methods (Baraff et al. 1998) which allowed significant speedup in the simulation of particle systems. These implicit integration methods were subsequently improved and tuned to allow good simulation performance, both in the context of fast interactive garment animation and accurate simulation of complex garments (Eberhardt et al. 2000; Hauth and Etzmuss 2003b; Volino and Thalmann 2005).

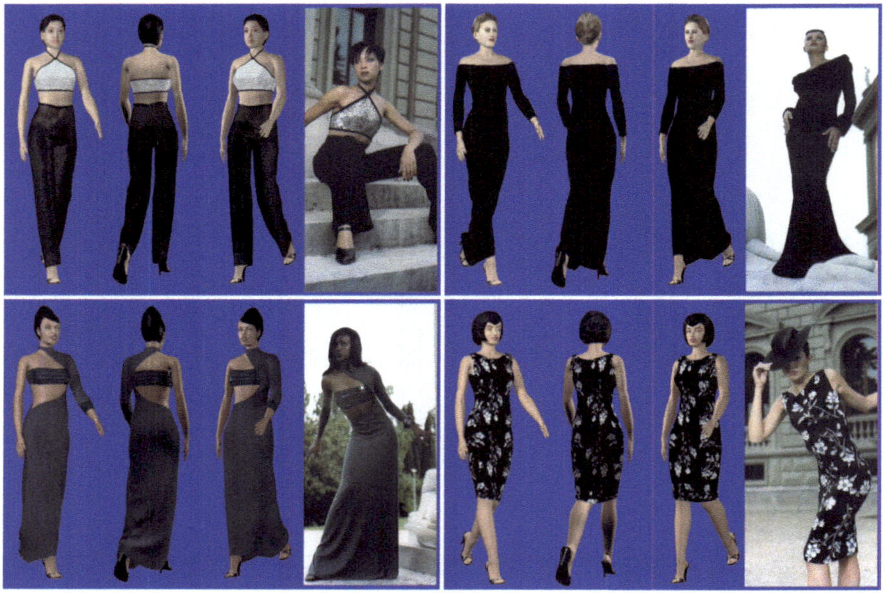

Fig. 3.4 Virtual fashion show models, and their real counterparts (Volino and Magnenat-Thalmann 1997)

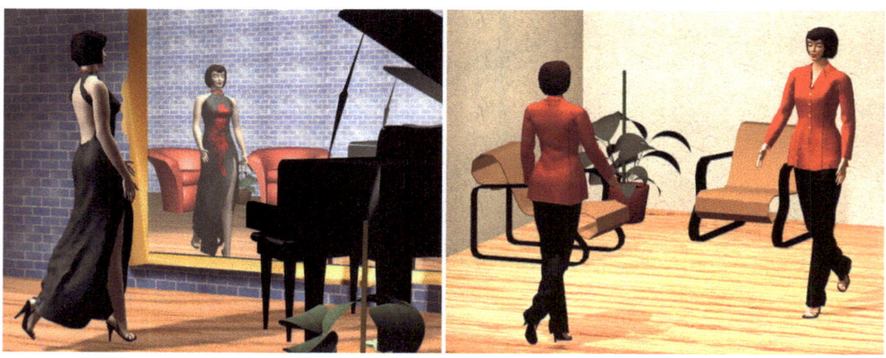

Fig. 3.5 Complex virtual garments

At the meantime, the accuracy of particle systems were has been highly improved, dropping the traditionally used spring-mass representations in favor of more complex representations derived from continuum mechanic representations, making then analogous to finite element representations (Etzmuss et al. 2003a) (Volino and Magnenat-Thalmann 2005). All these recent developments have led to the techniques described in the following sections (Fig. 3.5).

3.2 Measuring Physical Parameters

3.2.1 Introduction

Even very simple systems cannot be completely replicated with scientific methods, as it would be impossible to know the coordinates of all particle elements, at each time, their temperature, their movement and transformations. In scientific approaches, people are dependent on conceptual models, to reduce problems and questions to the essential.

Mechanical models approach reality by considering forces and impulses. Other influencing factors, necessary for a 100% identical imitation, are neglected. Mechanical models for virtual garment simulations represent the environment in which a virtual cloth is reproduced. At this the number of possibilities for different materials is infinite. On the other hand, to be able to simulate one specific fabric material, the precise virtual imitation of its real mechanical and physical characteristics is indispensable.

Regarding mechanics, fabrics are complex viscoelastic materials. Generally, materials can be divided into three main different types: solids, fluids and gases. A solid material, subjected to stress, recovers its original state as soon as the stress is removed. In contrast, if a fluid material is subjected to stress it flows and only gradually comes to rest when the force is removed. Materials such as textiles, which show characteristics of both, liquids and solids, are called viscoelastic materials (Askeland and Phulé 2005). Their simulation is not easy, as their behavior is difficult to describe and predict. Fabrics must have sufficient strength and at the same time they have to be flexible, elastic and easy to pleat and shape. Viscoelastic materials exhibit stress/strain comportment that is history and time dependent. The knowledge of the viscoelastic behavior of a material is based on empirical data from characterization experiments.

For fabrics, the research on mechanical properties has been driven for many decades by the need of a generalized, objectively measurable quality assessment. Therefore, important properties have been identified and their correlation has been studied. Investigations resulted in standardized fabric characterization experiments. Lately this research has been exploited for virtual simulations of textiles, because from the measured data, important input parameters for virtual simulations can be derived.

3.2.2 The Concept of Fabric Hand

The oldest known textiles (wool and cotton) date back to around 7,000 years ago and appeared with the invention of proficiencies such as spinning and weaving. In comparison to fabrics based on natural fibers, synthetic fibers are a relatively recent achievement. Only at the beginning of the twentieth century were the first full chemical fibers, the so-called "Synthetics", invented (Loschek 1995). Over the millennia the variety of textile materials increased continuously. Fabrics for different activities, climates or tendencies and trends have been developed to guarantee an optimal comfort of garments. With the development of new fibers (synthetics) and the continuous enhancement of new material structures, the variety of different fabric materials has become immense over the years and is still increasing (smart textiles). However, the development of such a variety of new fabric materials has led to an increasing difficulty in evaluating fabrics according their quality and suitability.

Each textile possesses specific characteristics, which are advantageous for some types of garments, but can be unfavorable for others, regarding comfort. Fabric characteristics are primarily influenced by the textiles raw material, yarn structures (degree of twist), planar structure (weave, knit) and finishing treatment. They can be either of physiological or aesthetical importance (Minazio 1995). For example synthetic fibers are easy to care for and keep their shape well, but do not conduct humidity well and lead easily to sweat (Fig. 3.6).

Aesthetical properties are the ones which are more subjective, complex and more difficult to grasp, for example firmness/smoothness, resistance to wrinkling

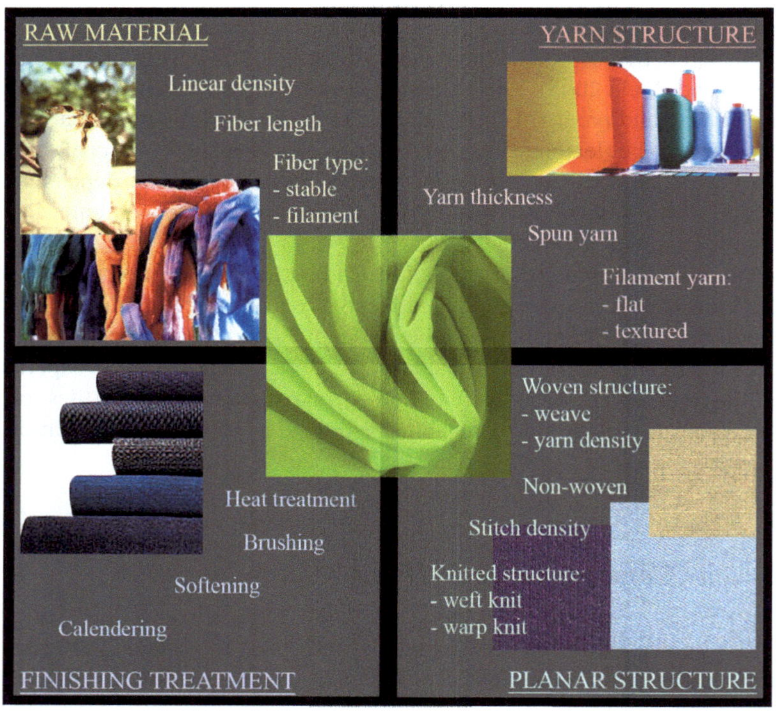
RAW MATERIAL
Linear density
Fiber length
Fiber type:
- stable
- filament
YARN STRUCTURE
Yarn thickness
Spun yarn
Filament yarn:
- flat
- textured
Woven structure:
- weave
- yarn density
Non-woven
Stitch density
Knitted structure:
- weft knit
- warp knit
PLANAR STRUCTURE
Heat treatment
Brushing
Softening
Calendering
FINISHING TREATMENT

Fig. 3.6 Scheme on influencing factors

or pilling resistance. The wrinkling of linen fabrics is a typical aesthetic fiber characteristic. The use of unsuitable or inferior fabrics is often the fundamental aspect that determines the success or failure of a textile product (Mäkinnen et al. 2005). Also the increasing automation of apparel manufacturing processes demands a more precise control of fabric characteristics (Zhou and Ghosh 1998). Thus, it became more and more important to judge textiles before any production process.

The concept of "fabric hand" was an important method of fabric assessment which was introduced by the apparel and textile industry. The term "fabric handle" or simply "handle" or "hand" is also used. Fabric hand refers to the total sensation, experienced when a fabric is touched or manipulated in the fingers. The attractiveness of a fabric's handle depends on its end use, as well as on possible cultural and individual preferences of the wearer (Minazio 1995). Fabric hand attributes can be obtained through subjective assessment or objective measurement.

3.2.2.1 Subjective Fabric Hand Assessment

Subjective assessment is the traditional method of describing fabric handle. Textiles are touched, squeezed, rubbed or otherwise handled by experts to judge their hand. The subjective assessment may thus be defined as a psychological reaction to the sense of touch (Mäkinnen et al. 2005). Disadvantages of the subjective hand assessment are on the one hand the varying sensitivity of people according to age, gender, skin hydration or cultural backgrounds in a tested population and on the other hand the difficulty of finding common standard expressions for specific hand sensations. Therefore, the organization AATCC (American Association of Textile Chemist and Colorists) has published guidelines for the generalization of the conditions during subjective hand evaluation (Website AATCC) (Figs. 3.7 and 3.8).

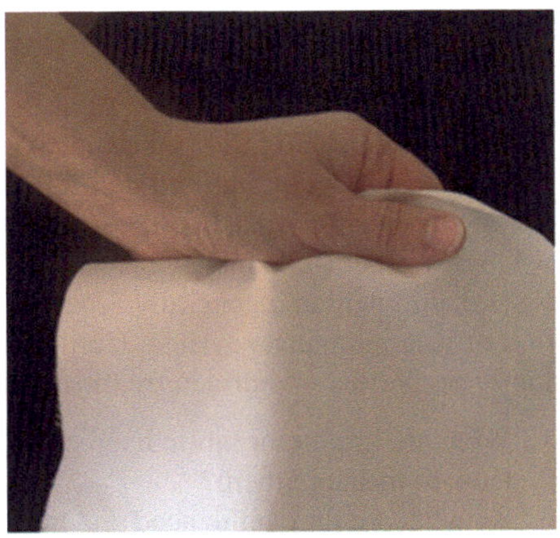

Fig. 3.7 Subjective fabric hand assessment

Fig. 3.8 Objective measurement

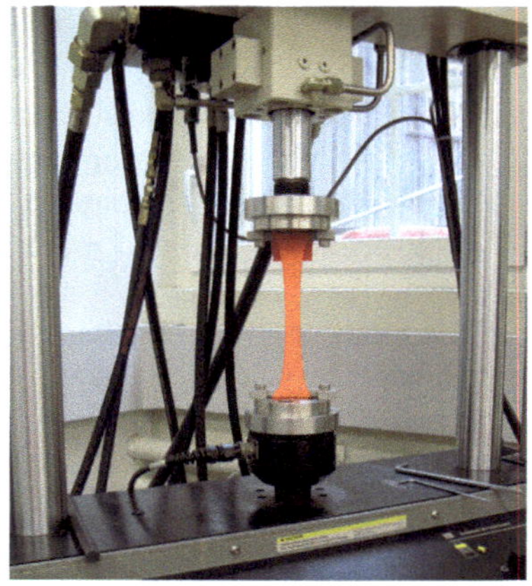

3.2.2.2 Objective Hand Measurements

Researchers have recognized the need to devise physical tests that analyze and reflect the sensation felt during subjective assessment and to describe the sensation of touching by a numerical value (Peirce 1930). Resulting objective assessments improved and standardized the communication on the abstract hand expressions and removed some of the "felt" subjectivity (Minazio 1995). During objective assessment, the fabric characteristics are measured with instruments and one "hand" value is calculated by relating the instrumental data. Important physical and mechanical properties are flexibility, compressibility, elasticity, resilience, density, surface contour (roughness, smoothness), surface friction and thermal character. These characteristics are the result of a broad fundamental research on fabric properties. Important standard measurement devices consist in the "Kawabata Evaluation System for Fabrics" (KES-f) and the "Fabric Assurance by Simple Testing" (FAST) method.

Fundamental Research

The first research on fabric mechanical properties dates back to Peirce in 1930, who can be seen as the pioneer in that field. In his first studies, he described a way of linking fabric properties in order to predict their behavior. However, until the 1980s, when Kawabata conducted his study on the standardization of objective hand assessment, neither a generally accepted definition of hand, nor an accepted definition of its components existed. Until then, the fundamental research on mechanical fabric properties was driven by three main questions:

1. What are important fabric hand characteristics?
2. How to measure them?
3. By what are they influenced and how are they related to each other?

1. What are important fabric hand characteristics?

The importance of fabric properties varied over time, depending on needs in manufacturing and the state of the art of fabric materials. On the one hand, until the 1960s, very little attention was given to the elasticity of fabrics. On the other hand, fabrics containing elastane did only exist from 1962 on, following the invention of synthetic materials (Website Dupont). In the beginning of the fundamental research the focus was on the stiffness parameter (or bending, flexibility). In comparison to other characteristics, stiffness was an important tailoring and drape aspect and also probably the property, which was the most difficult to understand. Also Peirce considered stiffness properties, such as bending length and flexural rigidity, as the most important properties regarding hand (Peirce 1930). After 1960, researchers 2009also focused more on fabric buckling and shear properties. Other fabric hand properties such as compressibility, friction or the surface contour were easier to grasp and describe and thus, their investigation seemed to be less important.

2. How to measure them?

Researcher thought of different experiments for the measurement of each single fabric property. Tensile measurements are designed to return the fabric elongation for a corresponding force. Bending measurements can be classified in two main categories. The first group measures the bending deformation of a fabric under its own weight. Within this category, Peirce developed several stiffness testing methods. The most important one was the Cantilever method, which uses the engineering principles of beam theory. A fabric is moved forward to project as a cantilever from a horizontal platform. As soon as the leading edge of the fabric reaches an angle of 41.5° to the horizontal platform, the bending length is measured. The principle of this method is used in the FAST method. Apart from the Cantilever method, folded loop methods have been invented, where the fabric is fold back on itself and the height of the loop measured (Figs. 3.9–3.11).

The second group of bending measurements is designed to return the moment-curvature relationship by measuring forces or moments. In 1957, Isshi (Isshi 1957) developed the predecessor of Kawabata's bending testing apparatus, which is based on that principle. A fabric is fixed between two clamps and the specimen is bent in

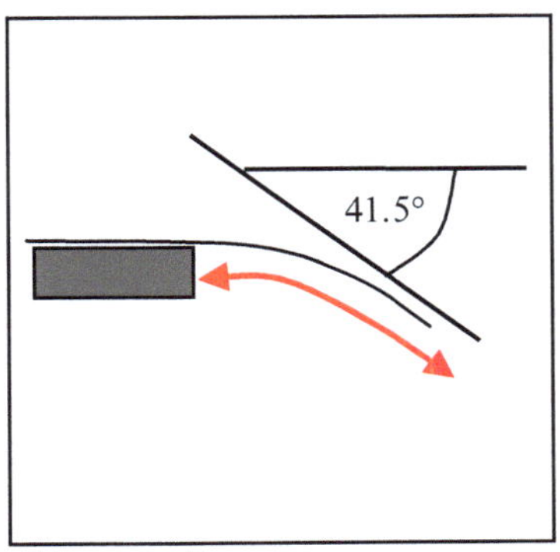

Fig. 3.9 Cantilever principle. Group 1

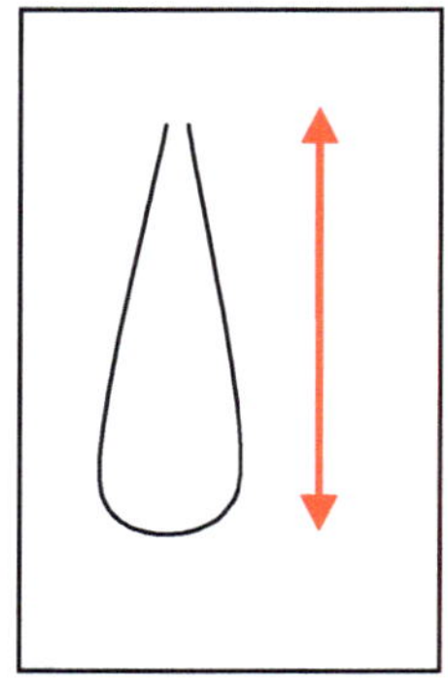

Fig. 3.10 Loop method. Group 1

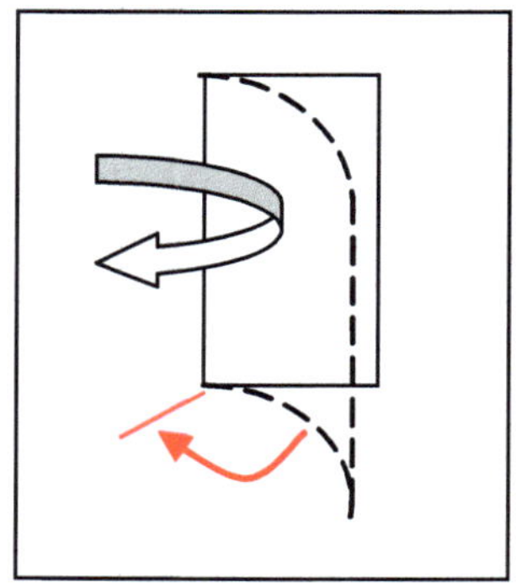

Fig. 3.11 Moment-curvature method. Group 2

an arc of constant curvature and the curvature changes continuously. The curvature is returned by a pointer, which is fixed on the moving clamp.

In 1951, Abbott compared five different objective stiffness measurement devices with subjective assessment: Cantilever (Peirce), Heart loop (Peirce), Schiefer Flexometer, Planoflex, and Drapometer. Results indicated a significant correlation in four of the five methods. Peirce Cantilever was detected to return the closest results to subjective stiffness assessments (Abbott 1951).

In 1961, Behre, Lindberg and Dahlberg conducted an important threefold study on the relationship of fabric shear, buckling properties and garment appearance. This research contributed a lot to today's standard measurement methods, even their analysis was simplified by treating fabrics as thin plates and assuming isotropic behavior. Behre in 1961 proposed two alternative methods for measuring shear properties. He analyzed the stress distribution in a fabric sample, subjected to shear and used the results to construct a shear tester for routine testing. He described the relation of shear to the extension-compression in the bias direction of a woven fabric, as well as that a sample subjected to shear can be regarded as a cantilever, where the height is much larger than the width. For his shearing experiments, the measurements have been taken at a maximum force and the angle is measured (Figs. 3.12–3.14).

3. By what are they influenced and how are they related to each other?

During measurement, each fabric property is treated independently, whereas in reality all fabric characteristics are somehow related. Thus, measurements allow the characterization of single properties, but to really understand the behavior of an entire fabric it is important to know the mutual influences of the single properties to each other.

Cooper (Cooper 1960) tried to derive the fabric stiffness property from fiber stiffness properties in studying their complex relationship. His studies revealed that regarding fabric stiffness, it is important whether the fiber inside the yarn or the yarn inside the fabric can move freely. The free fiber movement is basically inhibited by the fabric structures or finishing. For fabrics with a tight structure, the stiffness increases towards that of a solid sheet of material, which state is however never

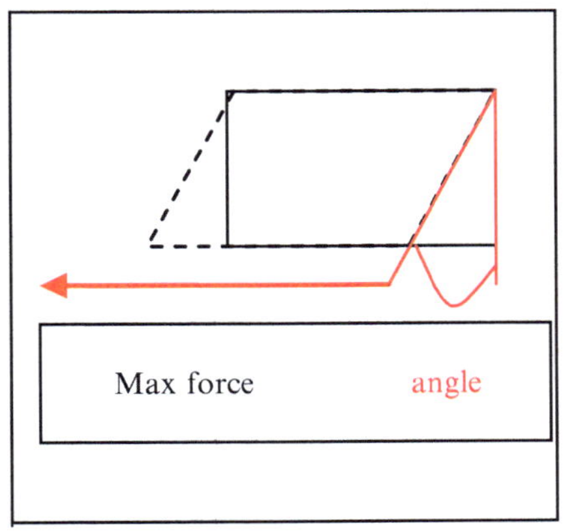

Fig. 3.12 Angle force method

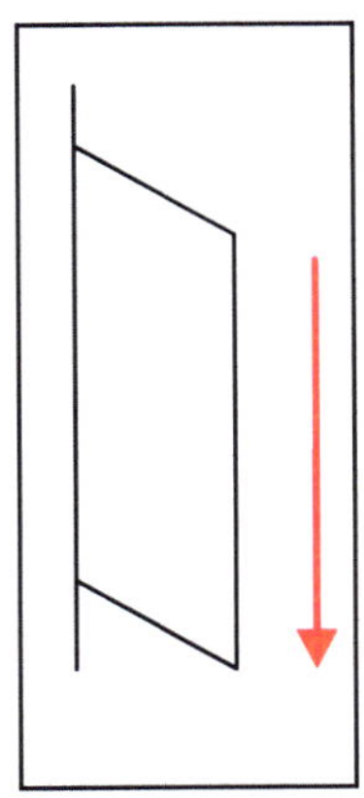

Fig. 3.13 Shear seen a cantilever

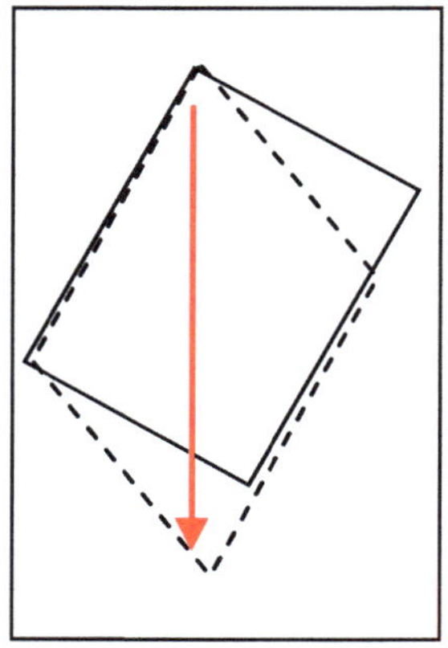

Fig. 3.14 Shear in 45°

reached in practice. Weave differences are also important, especially the floats/satin, as with floats the fabric is looser.

Livesey (Livesey and Owen 1964) later stated that the correlation of inter-fiber friction and fiber movement is the major cause of the nonlinear bending behavior.

In 1966 Grosberg also conducted research on the nonlinear behavior of bending. He found out that due to the frictional restraints, the fabric bending behavior is initially indeed nonlinear, but that with increased loads, the behavior becomes linear. He showed that the Cantilever is suited for a rapid measurement of the parameters of cloth with small frictional restraint, while the buckling method is more suitable for rapid measurement of cloth with large frictional restraints (Grosberg and Swani 1966).

In the third part of their study, Lindberg and Dahlberg demonstrated that there is a linear relationship between bending stiffness and the buckling load and that there is also a relationship between the formability in the bias direction and the shear angle of a fabric (the highest formability of a fabric is generally in the bias direction). However, they found that there was no relationship between bending stiffness and shear angle. They invented the drawing of "fabric maps", considering bending stiffness and shear angle. The character of a material depends on its position on the map. FAST later uses a similar concept for their fabric "fingerprints" (Behre 1961; Dahlberg 1961; Lindberg and Dahlberg 1961).

In 1961, Cusick discovered the relationship between complex bending and the shear property. Cusick was better known for his studies on fabric drape. However, shear is an important influencing property on fabric drape. Cusick stated that because of the low flexural rigidity of fabrics (compared to other materials), a woven fabric may be bent into single curvature without any shear deformation, but if a fabric is bent into double curvature or more complex curvature, then shearing occurs. For his studies, he performed a series of experiments, where the fabric is sheared for two cycles in reversed directions until the fabric is observed to start to buckle. Later Kawabata adopted this method, but standardized it to a maximum shear angle of 8° (Cusick 1961,1965, 1968; Peirce 1937) also was the pioneer for the prediction of fabric properties with statistical methods, in order to reduce the number of time consuming characterization experiments. Therefore, he described the fabric structures with mathematical forms and tried to discover quantitative relations between fabric properties of general validity, by assuming simple geometrical forms and idealized characteristics of materials.

In 1985, Li developed a model for predicting shear buckling that combined the anisotropic characteristics of the fabric with bending stiffness properties (Li 1940).

Recently, researchers worked on the relation and prediction of fabric handle parameters through the help of so-called "neural fuzzy networks" (Hui 2004).

Kawabata (KES-f) (Kawabata 1980)

In the 1970s, Kawabata conducted research on mechanical fabric properties; however, his main achievement was the concentration of the so far obtained fundamental knowledge on fabric mechanics in one standardized fabric characterization methods. Since, his achievements represent the most wide spread and well-known method for the objective assessment of fabric hand. Until then, fabric hand experts in factories, sales engineers or consumers executed fabric hand assessments subjectively without any common concept or definition of hand, in spite of the importance.

Kawabata's standardization study was twofold. On the one side he organized an expert committee with different people from the apparel industry, who assessed traditionally in total around 1,500 different fabric materials. According to the expert team, a "good" hand meant for example that to the touch the fabric is extremely smooth and both, stiffness and fullness/softness are moderate. The main goal of the expert team was to identify the most important hand expressions and to relate these touch sensations to measurable fabric properties. Kawabata then developed a method for relating the measured data in a way, so that 16 characteristic values such as linearity, shear stiffness, bending rigidity, mean value of the friction coefficient, etc. could be calculated. Out of the 16 characteristic values, one single "good" or "poor" hand feeling is derived. This part of Kawabata's studies can be seen as the standardization procedure.

Besides his studies on the standardization of objective fabric hand assessment, Kawabata went on with research on mechanical and physical fabric properties. This part of research was driven by the question of how a broad variety of fabrics should be measured in the same way so that the obtained data represents a significant statement about that textile. When a fabric is touched and squeezed during subjective hand assessment, only small forces occur. For example, no fabric would break during this manipulation. For this reason, Kawabata designed his measurement standard for small deformation region. In conclusion, Kawabata considered six measurement blocks to obtain all necessary properties for the calculation of hand:

Group 1: Tensile property
Group 2: Bending property
Group 3: Surface property

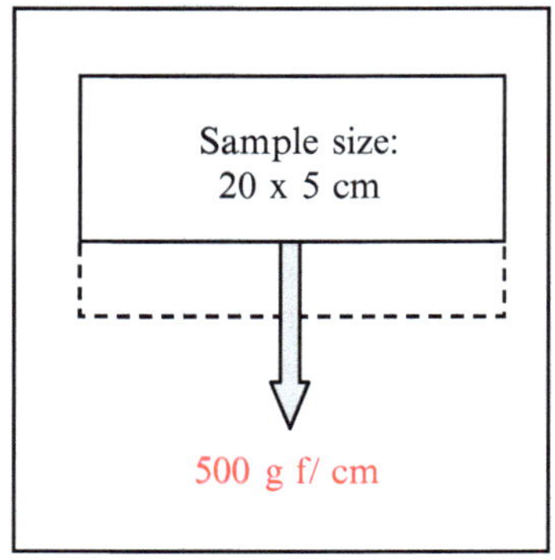

Fig. 3.15 Tensile measuring scheme

Group 4: Shearing property
Group 5: Compressional property
Group 6: Weight and thickness

Group 3 and 6 are physical properties and are indirectly related to mechanical properties, for example weight and thickness influence bending. In 1980 the machines were improved and named KES-FB, which consists of only four machine blocks:

- KES-FB 1 = Tensile and shearing test

Tensile deformation is applied along the length. The specimen size is 5 cm length to 20 cm width. The strain in the width direction becomes approximately zero because the force is applied to the long sides of a rectangular specimen. This type of deformation is also called "strip biaxial deformation". After the tensile force attains at Fm = 500 g f/cm, the recovery process is recorded. The tensile and shear tests can be conducted with velocities of either 0.1 or 0.2 mm/s (Fig. 3.15).

Characteristic values are:

LT: Linearity
WT: Tensile energy per unit area ($gf*cm/cm^2$)
RT: Resilience (%) (To which degree the fabric recovers, after the release of the force)

These characteristic values are defined by:

$$LT = WT / WOT,$$

$$WT = \int 0\ \varepsilon m\ Fd\ \varepsilon\ \left(gf * cm/cm^2\right)$$

$$RT = (WT' / WT) * 100$$

where:

WOT = Fm ε m/2 (area surrounded by dotted line in Fig. 3.16)

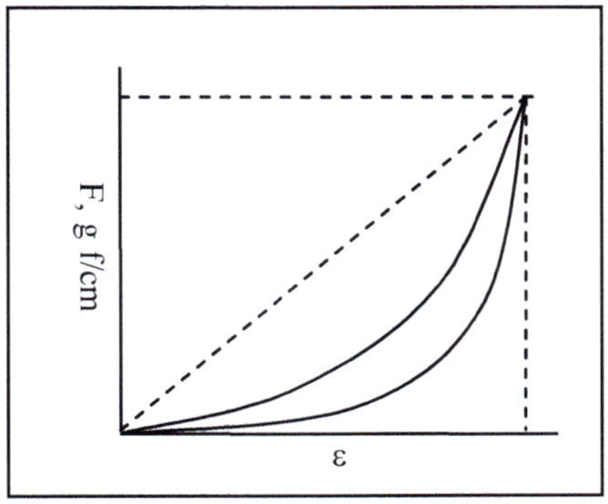

Fig. 3.16 Tensile hysteresis envelope

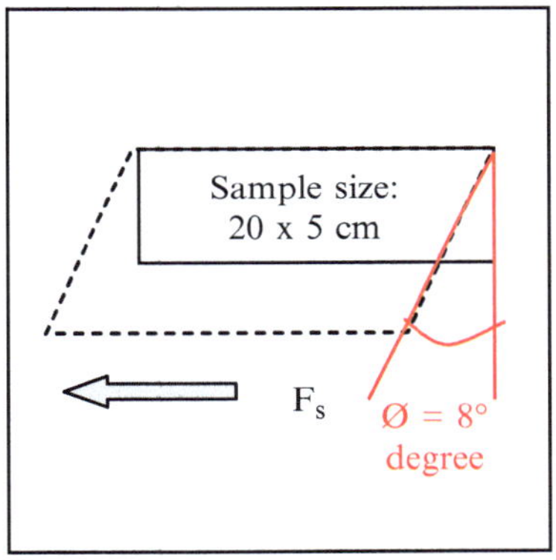

Fig. 3.17 Shear measurement scheme

F: Tensile force per unit width (gf/cm)
E: Tensile strain (ε has not % unit but is a dimensionless quantity)
Fm and εm: Maximum values of F and ε
W` = ∫ 0 ε m F`d ε (recovering energy per energy unit area)
F`: Tensile force in recovering process

In a more recent study of the relaxation phenomena of fabrics containing elastane yarns, a modification of the KES-FB standard from 500 g f/cm to 490.5 Nm^{-1} is recommended for fabrics containing elastane, as their relaxation is different from those, without any elastane (Gersak et al. 2005).

For shearing a constant tension along the direction, orthogonal to shearing force of W = 10 gf/cm is applied. This deformation should overlap initial biaxial tensile and shear forces. Shear properties are obtained by shearing the same specimen in 8° in one direction, then moving it back to the origin and shearing in the opposite direction until 8° is reached. Applied forces are recorded (Figs. 3.17 and 3.18).

Characteristic values are:

G: Shear stiffness (gf/cm * degree)
2 HG: Hysteresis at shear angle Ø = 0.5° (gf/cm)
2 HG5: Hysteresis at shear angle Ø = 5° (gf/cm)

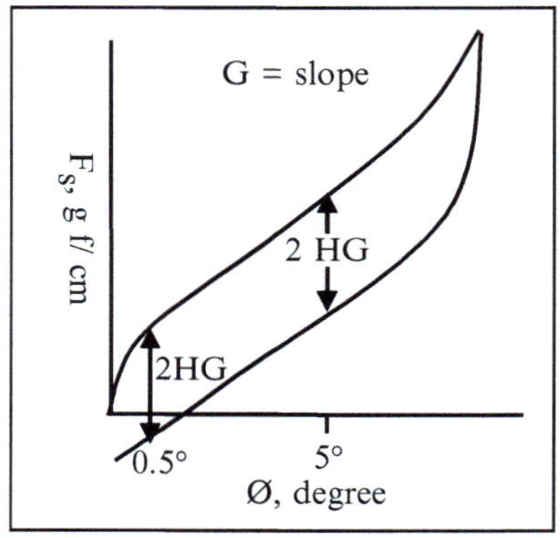

Fig. 3.18 Shear hysteresis envelope

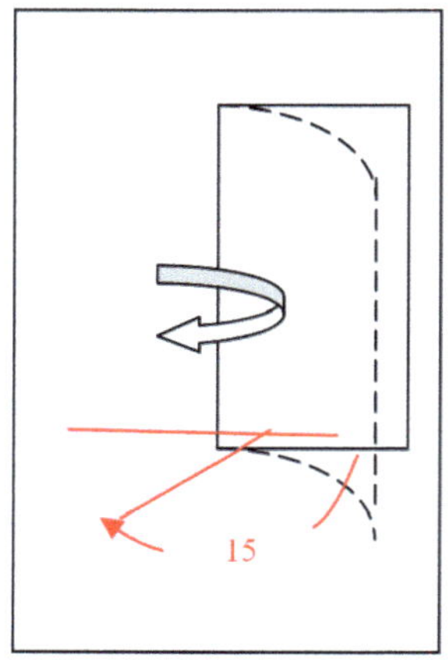

Fig. 3.19 Bending measurement scheme

G is defined as the (shear force per unit length) * (shear angle). G can also be defined as the slope of Fs – Ø between Ø = 0.5° and 5°. If the curve is not linear in this region, the mean slope over this region is taken. For fabrics with a non-symmetric weave structure, the curves are different between positive and negative regions. In this case, the measurement of both regions is necessary.

- KES-FB 2 = Pure bending test

Kawabata measures bending with an apparatus that bends the whole sample in an arc of constant curvature, where the curvature is changed continuously. This allows the detection of the relationship between bending momentum and curvature. The bending tester measures the forces to bend the specimen up to 150° followed by the opposite direction. (K = –2.5 cm^{-1} and 2.5 cm^{-1}). Specimen size is 20 cm by 1 cm width. The rate of curvature change is 0.50 cm^{-1}/s (Fig. 3.19).

Characteristic values are:

B: Bending rigidity per unit length (gf cm^2/cm)
2 HB: Momentum of hysteresis per unit length (gf cm/cm)

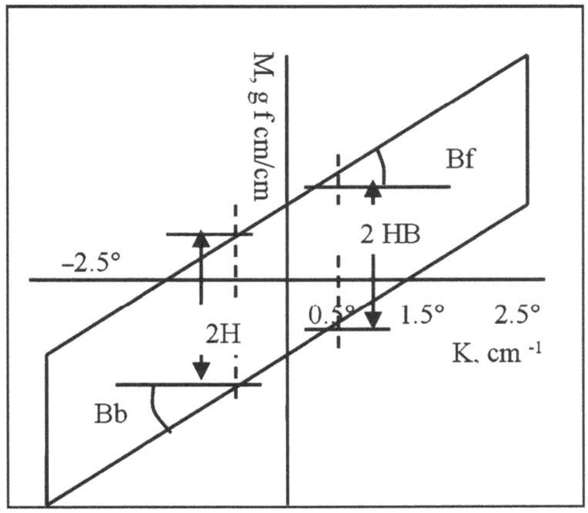

Fig. 3.20 Bending hysteresis envelope

B is defined by the slope between K = 0.5 and 2.5 for Bf and between K = –0.5 and –1.5 for Bb. Four types of bending are important: Face (Bf), Back (Bb) for weft and warp.

2HB means two times HB and can be measured as the hysteresis as in Fig. 3.20). It is taken between K = 0.5 and 1.5 for HBf and between K = –0.5 and –1.5 for HBb. For the calculation of the hand value, the mean value of all four is taken. However, depending on the interest, only one value can be taken.

- KES-FB 3 = Compressional test

Compression tests measure the compressibility of a textile as well as physical characteristics such as thickness and weight. Thickness in mm is measured with a fixed pressure of P = 0.5 gf/cm^2. Weight is expressed as mass density (mg/cm^2).

- KES-FB 4 = Surface test

Within the surface tests, friction is measured with piano-wire. The piano-wire is used under a constant force of 10 g and frequency is 30 Hz. The sample size for surface tests is 20 × 3.5 cm.

The sampling rates in various measurements can be fixed differently according to requirements. For example for bending, the sample rate is 20 Hz and in surface profiles and friction it is 1 kHz.

Characteristic values are:

MIU: mean value of the coefficient of friction
MMD: mean deviation of the coefficient of friction
SMD: mean deviation of surface roughness
Where MIU and SMD are:

$$\mathrm{MIU} = 1/X \int 0 \times \mu \, dx$$

$$\mathrm{MMD} = 1/X \int 0 \times |\mu - \mu'| \, dx$$

$$\mathrm{SMD} = 1/X \int 0 \times |T - T'| \, dx$$

Where:

μ: frictional force
x: displacement of the contactor on the surface of the specimen
X: 2 cm is taken in this standard measurement
T: Thickness of the specimen at position x, the thickness is measured by the contactor
T`: Mean value of T

- FAST (Minazio 1995; De Boos and Tester 1994)

Although Kawabata's objective assessment method is precise from a mechanical point of view, it was not widely adopted by the textile and clothing industry. Many companies still used the subjective evaluation to assess fabric hand. The main reason for this situation was the repetitive and lengthy process of measurements and expensive equipment. In the late 1980s CSIRO Division of Wool Technology in Australia realized the importance of a simpler and cheaper alternative to KES-f and developed the FAST -method. SiroFAST characterization standard resulted in three instruments and one test method:

- SiroFAST – 1: Compression Meter

Compression is taken at two loads: 2 and 100 g/cm². The measurements are taken once and are then repeated after the fabric has been relaxed with steam. Original surface thickness and the released surface thickness are measured and can be used to assess the stability of the finish of the fabric under garment manufacturing conditions such as pressing and steaming.

- SiroFAST – 2: Bending meter

This instrument measures the bending length using the cantilever bending principle. From the bending length, the bending rigidity is measured. Bending is measured in three directions, machine, cross and bias (45°) direction.

- SiroFAST – 3: Extensibility meter

The Extensibility meter measures the extensibility of a fabric under three different loads (5, 20 and 100 g/cm width). These loads are chosen to simulate the level of deformation that a fabric is likely to undergo during garment manufacture. This device is also used to measure the bias extensibility of the fabric (= shear) under a low load (5 g/cm width). Bias extensibility is not used directly but rather it is used to calculate shear rigidity.

In addition, formability parameters can be derived from SiroFAST-3 measurements in conjunction with data from SiroFAST-2.

- SiroFAST – 4: Dimensional stability test

The dimensional stability test is a procedure for measuring dimensional properties of fabrics such as hygral expansions and relaxations of fabrics (important for wool).

Parameters which describe the resistance to deformation, such as tensile (extensibility), bending (bending rigidity) and shear (shear rigidity) are considered as the most important. Similar to Kawabata, all measurement devices are designed for small deformation regions. FAST – 1, 2, 3 test samples must be 15 × 5 cm. The force is applied on the smaller side of the specimen (5 cm) and acts only on 10 cm length, as the fabric is hold by clamps. The same samples are used for all of the tests. (For Kawabata, multiple samples are needed.) About six to ten different fabrics can be measured in 1 day. The measuring conditions are the same as for the Kawabata equipment: room temperature should be 20° and room humidity should be 65%. The test results are summarized in the FAST control chart, also called fingerprint.

Other Measurement Systems

Today, in the community of garment physiology and engineering, there are discussions about the suitability of existing measurement and garment evaluation methods. Most knowledge and methods date back to the 1970s and 1980s, where the textiles have been quite different from today. The assessment methods have to be adapted to new fabric materials, which possess different characteristics. One new generation measurement method is the FAMOUS system.

- FAMOUS – Fabric automatic measurement and optimization universal system

The general understanding of the current provision of equipment, following the extensive scientific and industrial use of the last 20 years is that the KES-f is regarded as a scientific device for research and FAST as a simplified alternative device for industrial use (Stylios 2005). Results of KES-f are precise but the measurement equipment is expensive and the testing procedures are time consuming. FAST is a cheaper alternative to KES-f, but the tests are limited to one load only, which is measured and does not provide a complete stress/strain profile. FAMOUS tries to offer a new measurement method, consisting of only one apparatus to reduce equipment costs. The second aim is to reduce the time and complexity of the measurement procedure and to increase the accuracy of the measurements, compared to existing methods. During measurement of a textile, only one sample of 20 × 20 cm is needed and this is placed on the machine. The order of measurements is as follows: Flexural rigidity, shear, surface, compression and tensile. A complete suite of measurements takes only 5 min (Stylios 2005).

- Instron Tensile Tester (ITT)

Tensile and shear properties can also be measured with alternative measurement devices such as the Instron Tensile Tester (Website Instron). These alternative devices are often used to test breaking loads of materials and fabrics. Small and large deformation regions can be measured.

3.2.3 *Fabric Drape*

Fabric drape is not a mechanical or physical hand property but an important aesthetical parameter of fabrics. Drape determines the adjustment of clothing to the human silhouette and is defined as the extent to which a fabric will deform whilst hanging under its own weight. The ability of a fabric to drape can be seen as the main distinction between textiles and other sheet materials. An important measurement device is the drapemeter, where a circular piece of fabric is placed over an inner circular disc and an outer annular disc. During the drape test, the sample is placed over the two discs and the outer annular disc is lowered gradually, allowing the fabric to drape inside (Figs. 3.21 and 3.22).

Cusick developed a drapemeter, where one characteristic value, the drape coefficient, is calculated for a tested fabric. The drape coefficient can be defined as the percentage of the area of the annular ring covered by a vertical projection of the draped fabric (Cusick 1968). A high drape coefficient means that there is little deformation and vice versa.

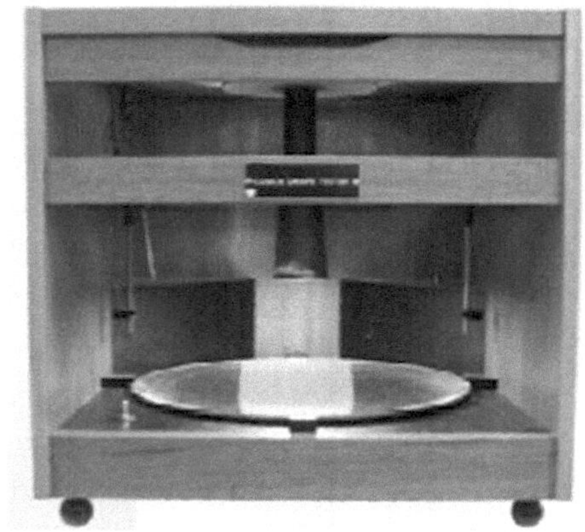

Fig. 3.21 Drapemeter

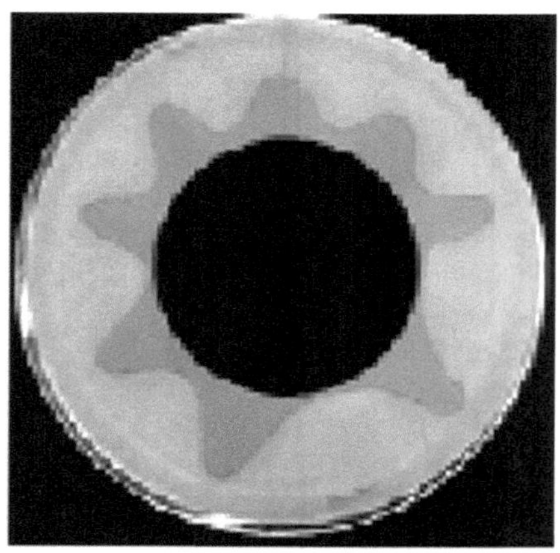

Fig. 3.22 Output picture (Kenkare and May-Plumlee 2005)

$$\text{Drape coefficient} = \frac{\text{Shaded area} - \Pi\left(r^2\right)*100}{\Pi\left(R^2 - r^2\right)}$$

R is the radius of the outer and r the radius of the inner circle.

Other research has been conducted to study the relationship of drape to corresponding fabric mechanical properties. Cusick found that drape is strongly related to bending rigidity and shear stiffness (Cusick 1965). Later on it was thought that the fabric weight and bending modulus are the most influencing factors on fabric drape. Collier claimed that shear and shear hysteresis are the most important influences on the fabrics drape characteristics (Collier et al. 1991).

Leapfrog (Website Leapfrog) is a large European project, which aim is to automate the entire clothing production chain with the help of new technologies. One goal of the project is the prediction of mechanical fabric properties out of drape characteristics, as fabric drape is faster, easier and cheaper to measure than precise mechanical properties. Thus, in the future, only the drape of new textiles should be recorded and mechanical parameters allocated. The FAST method and the Drapemeter have been used for this research. Correlations between the drape and mechanical parameters have been studied. However, no significant correlations between the fabric drape and the mechanical parameters have been found, except for the bending property and weight.

3.2.4 Mechanical and Physical Fabric Properties in Virtual Simulation Systems

Since the late 1990s, researchers focus on cloth simulation methods, where measured physical and mechanical parameters of fabrics constitute important input parameters for realistic virtual imitations of real textiles.

The first application of mechanical cloth simulations appeared in 1987 with the work of Terzopoulos. At that time, no measured mechanical and physical fabric properties had been used as input parameters. Parameters for different fabric behavior were set arbitrarily, as for instance rubber (Terzopoulos et al. 1987). Subsequent methods such as (Lafleur et al. 1991; Carignan et al. 1992; Baraff et al. 1998), focused on the accurate modeling of the simulation systems. The precision of input parameters was neglected, as algorithms were not yet able to handle accurately the complex behavior of fabrics. Fabric properties were simplified by linear and isotropic behavior assumption.

Later, some simulation systems (Breen et al. 1994; Bottino et al. 2001; Collier et al. 1991; Volino and Magnenat-Thalmann 2005), tested the versatility of their applications with empirical data from standard fabric characterization experiments such as KES-f. (Eberhardt et al. 1996; Eberhardt and Weber 1999; Eberhardt and Weber 1997), used energy potentials and included both the loading and unloading KES data. Collier also used the Drapemeter for the derivation of input parameters. KES-f data was used for tensile data and shear.

In the German Research project "Virtual Try On", the properties of fabric combinations and processed materials, such as fused or interlined textiles, are measured for the first time. Therefore the KES-f method has been used (Website Hohenstein).

The aim of European project Haptex is the virtual simulation of the touch of fabrics in real-time. The KES-f method is used for the determination of fabric input parameters (Website Haptex).

3.3 Physical Simulation of Cloth

3.3.1 Introduction

Garment simulation and animation is at the crossroad of many technologies, which by essence involve physically-based mechanical simulation for reproducing adequately the shape and the motion of the garment on the virtual body, as well as collision detection for modeling the interactions between the garments and the body. These are combined using advanced numerical methods and algorithms aimed at obtaining the best compromise between computational performance, accuracy and robustness in the process of cloth design, simulation and animation (Fig. 3.23).

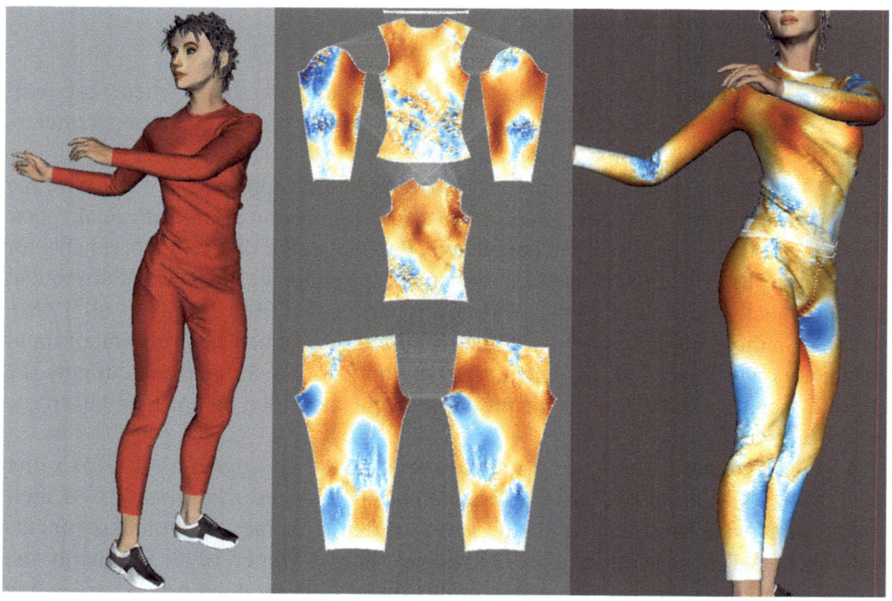

Fig. 3.23 Accurate mechanical models linked to efficient numerical methods are required for obtaining simulation systems efficient enough for virtual prototyping applications

3.3.2 Physical Properties of Cloth Materials

The mechanical properties of fabric material account for how it reacts to given stimuli, such as imposed deformations, constraints or force patterns. Experimental procedures, mainly based on tensile and bending tests, can be used to evaluate the mechanical behavior of cloth materials, which then needs to be expressed according to formalisms related to physics and mechanics.

In the following, we describe the concepts of tensile strain and stress, relating the in-plane deformation of 2D materials such as cloth. The relationship between strain and stress, which describes the behavior of the material, can have particular features which are then described. The same concepts may be applied to bending, describing the behavior in out-of-plane deformations (folds and wrinkles).

From the theory of elasticity (Timoshenko and Goodier 1970; Gould 1993), the internal tensile deformation of a surface is characterized by its *strain*, measured through a *strain tensor*, represented by three independent values $\boldsymbol{\varepsilon}_{\mathbf{uu}}$, $\boldsymbol{\varepsilon}_{\mathbf{vv}}$, $\boldsymbol{\varepsilon}_{\mathbf{uv}}$ related to the coordinate system (**U**, **V**) of the material. In dynamical systems, their rate is measured though their time derivatives $\boldsymbol{\varepsilon}_{\mathbf{uu}}'$, $\boldsymbol{\varepsilon}_{\mathbf{vv}}'$, $\boldsymbol{\varepsilon}_{\mathbf{uv}}'$. Meanwhile, the internal tensile forces are characterized by its *stress*, modeled accordingly using a *stress tensor* represented by three independent values $\boldsymbol{\sigma}_{\mathbf{uu}}$, $\boldsymbol{\sigma}_{\mathbf{vv}}$, $\boldsymbol{\sigma}_{\mathbf{uv}}$. The strain and stress values are related through the current energy per surface unit **w** of the material by the following relationships, for any deformation mode **m** among (**uu**, **vv**, **uv**):

$$\sigma_m = \frac{\partial w}{\partial \varepsilon_m} \tag{3.1}$$

The relationship between strain and stress defines the mechanical behavior of the material. In the most general context, this is expressed through the following strain-stress relationship:

$$\begin{aligned} &\sigma_{uu}\left(\varepsilon_{uu}, \varepsilon_{vv}, \varepsilon_{uv}, \varepsilon'_{uu}, \varepsilon'_{vv}, \varepsilon'_{uv}\right) \\ &\sigma_{vv}\left(\varepsilon_{uu}, \varepsilon_{vv}, \varepsilon_{uv}, \varepsilon'_{uu}, \varepsilon'_{vv}, \varepsilon'_{uv}\right) \\ &\sigma_{uv}\left(\varepsilon_{uu}, \varepsilon_{vv}, \varepsilon_{uv}, \varepsilon'_{uu}, \varepsilon'_{vv}, \varepsilon'_{uv}\right) \end{aligned} \tag{3.2}$$

An *isotropic* material behaves exactly identically whatever its orientation, and its strain-stress relationship does not depend on the orientation of the material coordinate system.

In the case of *linear viscoelasticity*, the strain-stress relationship can be expressed as a linear expression, the elastic and viscous stiffness of the material being represented as symmetric matrices **E** and **E'**:

$$\begin{bmatrix} \sigma_{uu} \\ \sigma_{vv} \\ \sigma_{uv} \end{bmatrix} = E \begin{bmatrix} \varepsilon_{uu} \\ \varepsilon_{vv} \\ \varepsilon_{uv} \end{bmatrix} + E' \begin{bmatrix} \varepsilon'_{uu} \\ \varepsilon'_{vv} \\ \varepsilon'_{uv} \end{bmatrix} \tag{3.3}$$

In the particular case of *isotropic linear elasticity*, the behavior of the material is only described with two parameters: The Young modulus **e** relates the stiffness of the material while the Poisson coefficient **ν** relates its transverse contraction upon extension. The corresponding matrix is the following:

$$E = \frac{e}{1-\nu^2}\begin{bmatrix} 1 & \nu & 0 \\ \nu & 1 & 0 \\ 0 & 0 & \frac{1-\nu}{2} \end{bmatrix} \tag{3.4}$$

While isotropic materials are well adapted for simulating homogeneous materials, cloth materials are mostly made of fibers which are oriented along particular directions. Thus, they are very unlikely to exhibit the same stiffness whatever the deformation direction (Fig. 3.24). Therefore, accurate representation of cloth materials requires anisotropic models. Among them, *orthotropic* models, which assume stiffness symmetry along orthogonal fiber directions (symmetric radial stiffness diagram), are only suited with cloth having orthogonal fiber orientations with symmetric weave patterns.

Since cloth materials often undergo large deformations, their behavior is rather nonlinear: Internal forces do not oppose much deformation as long as they remain low, but the stiffness quickly increases as soon as deformations become higher. From this behavior result the subtle deformability of these materials: They can move quite freely and drape nicely if left unconstrained, whereas they also retain their shape in tight situations. While linear approximations are often used for computational simplicity, accurate simulation of nice-looking cloth materials will highly benefit from nonlinear models.

Modeling adequately the strain-stress behavior is done through experimental procedures (typically tensile tests), followed by adequate approximations for fitting the requirements of the mechanical simulation scheme.

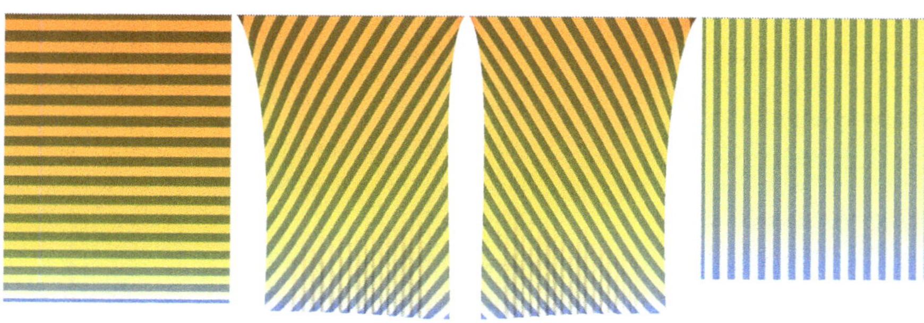

Fig. 3.24 Due to their fiber-based structure, cloth material exhibit anisotropic mechanical behaviors. For instance, their tensile stiffness varies according to the orientation

3.3.3 *Simulation Models*

3.3.3.1 Generalities on Mechanical Simulation

Mechanical simulation intends to reproduce virtual cloth surfaces with given parameters, which are expressed as strain-stress relationships (3.2). These can typically be described as curves, according to various degrees of simplification and approximation. While simple linear models can approximate these curves, more accurate models would model the curves with nonlinear analytic functions such as polynomials on interval-defined functions. Advanced models might also consider plasticity through the modeling of hysteresis in the curves, and viscosity by adding the deformation speeds in the expression of the internal forces of the fabric. Additionally to be considered is the density of the fabric (mass per surface unit).

The cloth also has to react to its environment. These interactions are obviously collisions with the environment objects which account for reaction and friction (most importantly for virtual garments, the body that wears the garment) as well as self-collision between various garment parts. Also comes gravity, which exerts a force proportional to the mass of the object, and thus a constant acceleration that pulls objects toward the floor. Advanced models might also consider aerodynamic forces, which in simple implementations are only viscosity forces related to the speed difference between the cloth and the surrounding air (wind speed), and in complex models result from an advanced computation of the motion of the surrounding air masses that interact with the cloth and other objects.

Whatever modeling is chosen for representing the behavior of the cloth material, additional equations are required to illustrate to fundamental laws of mechanics. Among them, *Newton's Second Law*, which relates the acceleration of objects to the force applied on it divided by its mass, is the most fundamental. Additionally, various *conservation laws* express the conservation of motion momentum within mechanical systems. These laws may be combined in integral of variational forms in many different ways for obtaining formulation that are suitable to the chosen mechanical simulation scheme.

Several different contexts have to be considered for garment simulation. Among them are *draping problems*, where the draping rest shape of a garment has to be computed on an immobile body, and *animation problems*, where the accurate garment animation has to be computed on a moving body. While a draping problem only needs the numerical solver to find the equilibrium of the equations as efficiently as possible using only elasticity laws, an animation problem requires the solver to compute accurately the evolution of the mechanical state along time, and necessitates the simulation of dissipative mechanical behaviors such as viscosity and plasticity. While a *quasistatic* solver which does not consider speed can be sufficient to deal with a draping problem, a *dynamic* solver simulating speed and inertia is necessary for an animation problem.

Combining the equations of material behavior with mechanical laws yields complex systems of mathematical equations, usually partial differential equations or other types of differential systems. Mathematics provides analytical solutions only for a limited class of simple equations, which would only solve very elementary situations involving simple models, and which have no interest for usual cloth simulation contexts. For complex cloth simulations, such solutions are not available, and the only practical solution is to implement numerical methods.

The numerical solution of a system of differential equations requires discretization, explicit computation of the physical values at precise points in space and time. *Space discretization* can either be accomplished through numerical solution techniques, such as in models derived from continuum mechanics, or be part of the mechanical model itself, as in particle system models. Usual discretizations consider polygonal meshes which allow convenient representation of the discrete mechanical representation. Mostly used are triangular meshes, regular or irregular, or regular square meshes. It is also possible to use meshes of curved patches (Spline, Bezier, subdivision) allowing reduction of the number of elements, or even implicit surfaces although they cannot be explicitly used for representing mechanical entities. *Time discretization* results from the numerical computation of a sequence of states during the time period. Interpolation of the successive states provides an approximation to the entire trajectory. There are several schemes for performing mechanical simulation, differing mainly on where the discretization takes place in the process. The two major families are:

- *Continuum mechanics*, which studies the state of material surfaces and volumes through quantities varying continuously in space and time. Each physical parameter of the material is represented by a scalar or vector value continuously varying with position and time. Mechanical and behavior laws can then be represented as a set of partial differential equations which hold throughout the volume of the material. While the mechanical representation of the object only depends on the model itself, numerical resolution often requires the discretization of the equations in the volume space.
- *Particle systems*, which discretize the material itself as a set of point masses ("particles") that interact with a set of "forces" which approximately model the behavior of the material.

The difference between these two schemes is that a particle system is a discrete model built on a related discrete surface representation, whereas continuum mechanics define a continuous model which is then discretized. This distinction is indeed blurred by the existence of accurate particle systems that accurately represent the actual behavior of the continuum media described as elements, becoming equivalent to continuum models where the media mass is condensed to discrete locations via the mass-lumping technique.

An overview of the various simulation systems available for cloth simulation can be found in (Nealen et al. 2005) (Fig. 3.25).

3.3.3.2 State-of-the-Art in Cloth Simulation Techniques

Early cloth simulation systems have been described as Particle Systems. They have always been of large interest in the field of cloth simulation, and more generally in

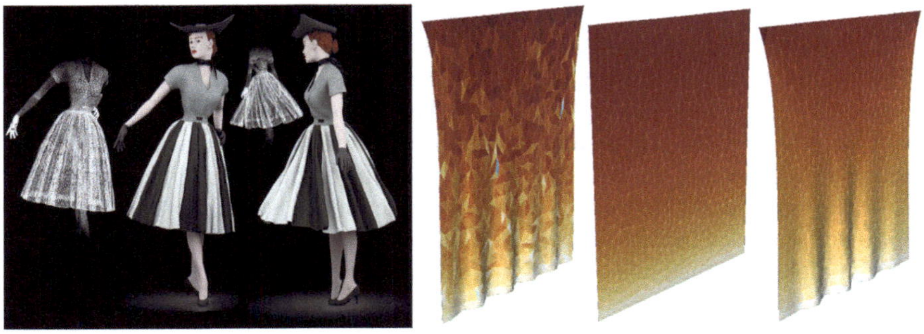

Fig. 3.25 Triangle meshes are the most common representation for complex garment objects (*left*). On them, fast, but inaccurate spring-mass particle systems can be implemented (*center*), as well as more accurate finite-element methods offering good representation of numerous mechanical behaviors (*right*)

the field of interactive mechanical simulation, as they offer a simple, intuitive and flexible way to model mechanical systems. Furthermore, they can be combined with a large range of numerical integration schemes, according to the relevant features of the simulation context (dynamic accuracy, convergence speed, fast and approximate simulation, robustness, etc.).

The first Particle Systems for cloth simulation were grid-based (Breen et al. 1994; Eberhardt et al. 1996), and already featured the simulation of nonlinear behavior curves through formulations that made them quite analogous to continuum-mechanics models. Their accuracy was however fairly limited for large deformations, and required quite long computation times. Faster models, based on spring-mass grids, have become popular since fast implicit numerical integration methods were used (Baraff and Witkin 1998), because they allow a simple expression of the Jacobian of the particle forces while requiring only simple computations (Desbrun et al. 1999; Meyer et al. 2001; Choi and Ko 2002). Combined with advanced implicit integration methods (Eberhardt et al. 2000; Hauth and Etzmuss 2001; Volino and Magnenat-Thalmann 2005), these simulation schemes have become popular for real-time and interactive applications. Unfortunately, spring-mass systems are quite unable to model surface elasticity accurately (Wang and Deravajan 2005). Although some techniques have been developed to match their parameters with those of the simulated material, they do not allow full discrimination between deformation modes (Bianchi et al. 2004), and they remain particularly inaccurate for anisotropic and nonlinear models. Particle Systems, as a whole, have inherited this reputation of inaccuracy from them.

On the other hand, Finite Elements have now acquired a good maturity for mechanical simulation. Their traditional field of application is elastic solid or shell modeling for mechanical engineering purposes, a context where linear elasticity and small deformations are the rules. These formulations are not so well adapted to very deformable objects such as cloth, and early attempts to model cloth using high-order elements (Eischen et al. 1996) led to impractically high computation times. However, it has been shown that the use of appropriate simplifications and efficient algorithms can make them usable in interactive graphics applications. Finite element methods proceed in several steps. First, a deformation tensor is expressed at each point inside the elements, based on the shape functions associated with the nodes. When linear shape functions are used, the elements are called first degree, otherwise they are called higher degree. The computer graphics community has mainly considered first-degree elements, bringing the best compromise between speed and accuracy in this context. Beside this, linearity can occur in two places in the finite element methods. The first one, which we call geometrical linearity, is related to the way strains are computed from node displacements. The simplest way is to use Cauchy's strain tensor, which is linear with respect to node displacements, and leads to the fastest computations. However, large rotations generate well-known bulging artifacts. The most general way is to use Green-Lagrange's strain tensor, which is nonlinear with respect to node displacements and handles large rotations without artifacts. The other linearity, which we call material linearity, is related to the physical properties of the material. Most models consider the linear Hooke's law relating strain and stress.

Numerous authors have attempted to speed up the computation times required for Finite Elements. Pre-inverting the linear system matrix (as done by (Desbrun et al. 1999) for Particle Systems) may speed up the computation (Bro-Nielsen and Cotin 1996; Cotin et al. 1999), but is only practical when the mechanical system is small enough. Condensing the dynamics on the boundary of a closed volume can reduce the number of unknowns to solve at each time step (James and Pai 1999). These precomputations are possible when the force-displacement relation is linear, which requires both geometrical and material linearity.

Large rotations have been handled in two different ways. The most straightforward is to use Green-Lagrange's nonlinear strain measurement, while keeping material linearity. This is called the Saint-Venant-Kirchhoff model, mainly used in volume simulation (Bonet and Wood 1997; O'Brien and Hodgins 1999; Zhuang and Canny 2000; Debunne et al. 2001; Hauth et al. 2003; Picinbono et al. 2003; Barbic and James 2005).

The force-displacement behavior of Saint-Venant-Kirchhoff models is less "intuitive", through the nonlinearity of their strain and stress tensors. Hence, their strain is not proportional to the deformation of the material, and the exerted force is not proportional to the stress. Actually, with strain-stress proportionality, the tensile force-deformation curve of such a material is cubic. However, their mathematical definition is indeed the most mathematically natural way of expressing strain and stress, and indeed the simplest, despite the nonlinearity.

The major drawback of this model is that it is not robust under large compression, since it is prone to collapse (Bonet and Wood 1997). Recently, a new approach has been proposed, where the strain tensor is factored as the product of a pure rotation with Cauchy's linear strain tensor aligned along the strain eigendirections (Muller et al. 2002; Hauth and Strasser 2004; Muller and Gross 2004; Irving et al. 2004; Nesme et al. 2005). This corotational approach has become very popular, as it combines the computational simplicity of using the linear Cauchy tensor with large deformations. This approach has been successfully used in cloth simulation (Etzmuss et al. 2003), but material nonlinearity was not considered. However, this approach requires additional computations for finding the eigendirections of the strain tensor and managing the rotations accordingly (particularly when dealing with anisotropic materials such as cloth). Furthermore, the effects of these direction changes are not taken into account in the Jacobian, which is therefore not perfectly accurate. Therefore, this method is mainly suited for simulating perfectly linear isotropic material with large deformations.

Meanwhile, cloth materials are usually not subject to large compression, as their very low bending stiffness would quickly allow them to buckle, quickly relaxing compression to lower values. Hence, the compression collapse behavior of Saint-Venant-Kirchhoff models is actually not an issue in this context. Also, we have no interest in simulating a perfectly linear force-deformation behavior for nonlinear cloth materials. Furthermore, avoiding rotations greatly simplifies the computation, particularly in the context of anisotropic cloth materials.

From this, Saint-Venant-Kirchhoff models can be considered as being a good cloth simulation model when it comes to simulate anisotropic and nonlinear cloth materials under large deformations, keeping the computation as simple as possible. Furthermore, they exhibit a cubic tensile force-deformation behavior which is already a more realistic approximation of real cloth materials than a linear force-deformation behavior when using proportional strain-stress laws. Hence, in the following section, we give an example of mechanical simulation method based on the Saint-Venant-Kirchhoff model, which is particularly well-suited for simulating the nonlinear behavior of cloth.

3.3.4 A Simple Method for Accurate Simulation of Nonlinear Cloth Materials

The goal is to be able to simulate very accurately complex cloth objects, such as complete garments on animated characters, with precise reproduction of the nonlinear mechanical behavior of cloth. The presented model addresses elasticity as well as viscosity, making the model suitable not only for draping applications, but also for dynamic motion computations which require mechanical damping.

The presented model is at the crossroad of Continuum Mechanics and Particle Systems: It considers interaction forces between particles which are the vertices of a triangle mesh, yet these forces are computed through an accurate evaluation of the surface mechanical state within each triangle mesh element. Therefore, it has significant analogies to first-order Finite-Elements approximated using mass lumping.

One of the directing ideas of this model is to consider that linearization may not be the best option for a computation scheme that aims at simulating mechanical properties that are in essence nonlinear. Indeed, this idea is the key consideration which allows us to design a highly accurate computation process for simulating accurately the nonlinear anisotropic tensile viscoelastic properties of cloth through a simple, highly streamlined and fast computation process, which can be combined to state-of-the-art numerical integration methods for optimal efficiency.

This computation scheme handles arbitrary triangle meshes which are typically generated from Delaunay triangulation. First, strains and stresses in these elements are expressed according to the nonlinear Green-Lagrange tensor, similarly as done for representing Saint-Venant-Kirchhoff materials. A key idea is to provide very simple expressions relating material strain to particle positions and material stress to particle forces, from which an accurate and efficient computation scheme can be obtained with very simple and streamlined algorithms. Furthermore, material strain rate are also related to particle velocities in the same manner, and this offers a new way to represent accurately material viscosity. All these developments are expressed without excessive abstract formalisms through "ready-to-implement" expressions allowing straightforward integration into computation algorithms.

The presented model only addresses tensile viscoelasticity, which deals with in-plane deformations. Meanwhile, bending elasticity deals with out-of-plane deformations (surface curvature), and its main visible effect is to limit fold curvature and wrinkle size. In the context of high-accuracy simulations, the presented tensile model can easily be complemented by a bending model using the schemes defined by (Grinspun et al. 2003) or (Volino and Magnenat-Thalmann 2006) (Fig. 3.26).

Starting from the most general anisotropic nonlinear viscoelastic strain-stress relationship (3.2) describing the mechanical behavior of the material is derived a simple computation scheme which can be applied to meshes made of arbitrary triangle elements, such as those obtained through Delaunay triangulation of arbitrary surfaces.

The algorithm processes triangle elements of the mesh describing the surface. Each element is described by its 2D parametric coordinates ($\mathbf{u}_a$, $\mathbf{v}_a$), ($\mathbf{u}_b$, $\mathbf{v}_b$), ($\mathbf{u}_c$,$\mathbf{v}_c$) of its vertices, referring to an orthonormal parametric coordinate system (in the context of cloth simulation, aligned to the weft and warp fiber directions). The current position of the deformed element is defined by the 3D world coordinates $\mathbf{P}_a$, $\mathbf{P}_b$, $\mathbf{P}_c$ of its vertices, and possibly velocity coordinates $\mathbf{P'}_a$, $\mathbf{P'}_b$, $\mathbf{P'}_c$. The weft and warp vectors are expressed in 3D world coordinates as $\mathbf{U}$ and $\mathbf{V}$, which are not

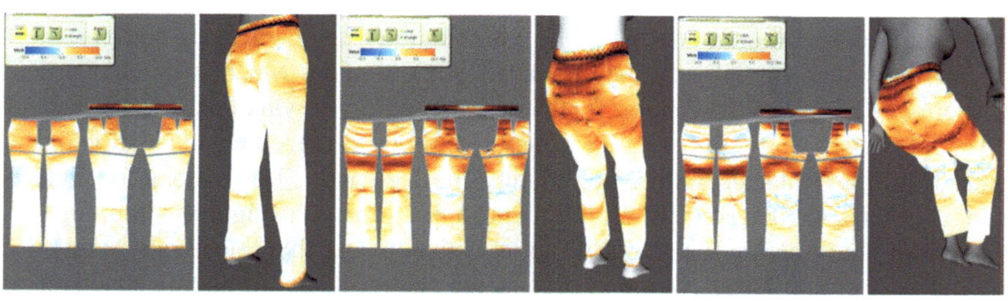

Fig. 3.26 The presented model offers enough accuracy for prototyping applications evaluating precisely the strain and stress state of the cloth, resulting from the nonlinear anisotropic behavior of the cloth

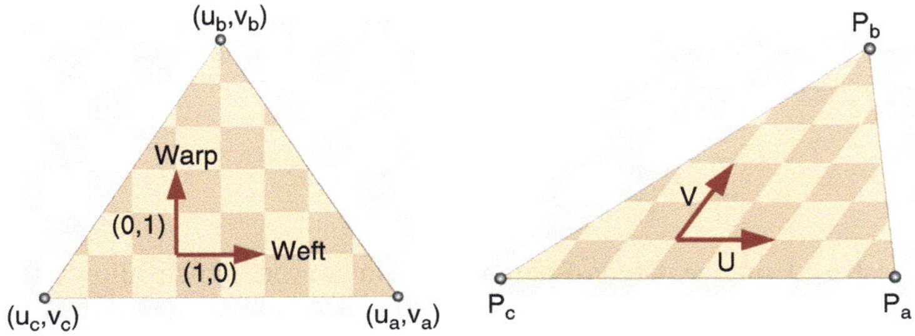

Fig. 3.27 The original shape of a triangle element is defined by its 2D parametric coordinates (*left*) while its current geometry is defined by the 3D world coordinates of its vertices (*right*)

necessarily orthonormal anymore because of material deformation (Fig. 3.27). In the following, these vectors will be used for measuring the deformation state of the element, as well as expressing any vector value related to the element in world coordinates.

The goal is to compute the deformation state of a triangle element directly from the positions of its vertices. To do this, we express the parametric coordinates the weft and warp orthonormal 2D vectors (1, 0) and (0, 1) as translation-independent weighted sums of the parametric coordinates of the three vertices ($\mathbf{u_a}$, $\mathbf{v_a}$), ($\mathbf{u_b}$, $\mathbf{v_b}$), ($\mathbf{u_c}$, $\mathbf{v_c}$). This leads to the following linear systems:

$$\begin{aligned} &\sum_i r_{ui}\, u_i = 1 && \sum_i r_{vi}\, u_i = 0 \\ &\sum_i r_{ui}\, v_i = 0 && \sum_i r_{vi}\, v_i = 1 \\ &\sum_i r_{ui} = 0 && \sum_i r_{vi} = 0 \end{aligned} \tag{3.5}$$

Solving these linear systems leads to the following weights, to be precomputed:

$$\begin{aligned} &r_{ua} = d^{-1}(v_b - v_c) && r_{va} = d^{-1}(u_c - u_b) \\ &r_{ub} = d^{-1}(v_c - v_a) && r_{vb} = d^{-1}(u_a - u_c) \\ &r_{uc} = d^{-1}(v_a - v_b) && r_{vc} = d^{-1}(u_b - u_a) \\ &d = u_a(v_b - v_c) + u_b(v_c - v_a) + u_c(v_a - v_b) \end{aligned} \tag{3.6}$$

During the simulation, these values are the weights for computing the current 3D vectors **U** and **V** directly as a weighted sum of the current vertex positions $\mathbf{P_i}$ (Fig. 3.27 right), as follows:

$$U = \sum_{i \in (a,b,c)} r_{ui}\, P_i \qquad V = \sum_{i \in (a,b,c)} r_{vi}\, P_i \tag{3.7}$$

When viscosity has to be considered in the context of dynamic simulations, the current evolution rates of the coordinate vectors **U'** and **V'** can be computed as well from the current vertex velocities $\mathbf{P'_i}$:

$$U' = \sum_{i \in (a,b,c)} r_{ui} P'_i \qquad V' = \sum_{i \in (a,b,c)} r_{vi} P'_i \tag{3.7'}$$

The model is based on the Green-Lagrange strain tensor, which allows the rotation-invariant description of internal surface strain in the context of large displacements. From this symmetric tensor, the weft warp and shear strain values, which respectively measure the elongation deformations along weft warp directions and the shear deformation between them, are computed as follows:

$$\begin{aligned} \varepsilon_{uu} &= \tfrac{1}{2}\left(U^T U - 1\right) \\ \varepsilon_{vv} &= \tfrac{1}{2}\left(V^T V - 1\right) \\ \varepsilon_{uv} &= \tfrac{1}{2}\left(U^T V + V^T U\right) \end{aligned} \tag{3.8}$$

Similarly, if viscosity is considered, the strain rate values are computed accordingly:

$$\begin{aligned} \varepsilon'_{uu} &= \left(U^T U'\right) \\ \varepsilon'_{vv} &= \left(V^T V'\right) \\ \varepsilon'_{uv} &= \left(U^T V' + V^T U'\right) \end{aligned} \tag{3.8'}$$

Having computed the strain state of the triangle surface, the stress state is obtained by using the strain-stress relationship (3.2) that characterizes the material of the surface.

The Green-Lagrange strain tensor is associated to the second Piola-Kirchhoff stress tensor through (3.1). The forces derive from energy (Bathe 1995). Hence, the forces $\mathbf{F_j}$ exerted on the vertex **j** are computed by derivation of the weft, warp and shear components of the total elastic energy **W** of the triangle relatively to the particle position $\mathbf{P_j}$. Since we assume linear deformation of the triangle element, we have uniform strain, stress and surfacic energy **w** over its surface of area **|d|/2** (3.6), and we have, for any **j** among (**a**, **b**, **c**):

$$F_j = -\frac{\partial W}{\partial P_j}^T = -\frac{|d|}{2}\frac{\partial w}{\partial P_j}^T = -\frac{|d|}{2}\left(\sum_{m \in (uu,vv,uv)} \sigma_m \left(\frac{\partial \varepsilon_m}{\partial P_j}^T\right)\right) \tag{3.9}$$

With explicit expression of the derivatives of the Green-Lagrange strain values (3.8) using (3.7) is obtained:

$$F_j = -\frac{|d|}{2}\left(\sigma_{uu}\left(r_{uj} U\right) + \sigma_{vv}\left(r_{vj} V\right) + \sigma_{uv}\left(r_{uj} V + r_{vj} U\right)\right) \tag{3.10}$$

Direct implementation of (3.7), (3.8), (3.2), (3.10) can be the basis of an accurate simulator integrated using explicit numerical time integration methods, such as Runge-Kutta (Eberhardt et al. 1996). In the context of implicit numerical integration methods (Baraff and Witkin 1998; Eberhardt et al. 2000; Hauth et al. 2001; Volino et al. 2005), the Jacobian, which is symmetric, can be extracted by derivation of (3.10) using (3.7) (3.8) and (3.2). The general topic of numerical integration is discussed in the next section.

3.3.5 *Numerical Integration*

The expression of the mechanical model for the global system leads to a differential system which has to be integrated for obtaining the evolution of the mechanical along time. In the context of particle systems, the differential system is typically an Ordinary Differential system containing which has the order of the number of degrees of freedom of the system (typically the number of particle coordinates). Except the very simple "school" problems considering elementary mechanical systems with one or two degrees of freedom and linear mechanical models, it is quite impossible to resolve analytically the differential equation systems describing the evolution of mechanical systems. Numerical resolution approximates the solution by a form of extrapolation from timestep to timestep, using the derivatives as evolution information. One of the main drawbacks of numerical simulation is the simulation error which accumulates from step to step. Optimized numerical methods can perform the numerical resolution by efficiently minimizing this error and the resulting simulation inaccuracy. This section will focus on these particular techniques that can be directly used with the mechanical model described in the previous section.

For dynamic mechanical simulation using particle systems, the problem can usually be reduced to the resolution of second order ordinary differential equation system where the variables are the particle positions along the evolving time. This problem is usually reduced to first-order through concatenation of position and velocity degrees of freedom. Solving the first-order ordinary differential equation obtained this way is a common problem of numerical analysis, well covered in the literature (Press et al. 1992). Numerous integration techniques exist, of different complexities and having optimal accuracy and efficiency in different contexts.

3.3.5.1 Explicit Integration Methods

Explicit integration methods are the simplest methods available for solving first-order ordinary differential systems. They consider the prediction of the future system state directly from the value of the derivatives. The most known techniques are the Runge-Kutta methods. Among them, the first-order Euler method, used in many early implementations, considers the future state as a direct extrapolation from the current state and the derivative. Higher order and more accurate methods also exist, such as the second-order Midpoint method, used for instance in (Volino and Magnenat-Thalmann 1995), and the fourth-order Runge-Kutta method, used for instance in (Eberhardt et al. 1996).

In typical cloth simulation situations, the fourth-order Runge-Kutta method has proven to be far superior to the second-order Midpoint method, which itself is significantly more efficient than the first-order Euler method. Although computationally more expensive than the Midpoint and Euler methods for each iteration, the larger timestep which can be used makes it worthwhile, especially considering the benefits in stability and accuracy. Increasing order, however, does not translate indefinitely into increasing precision. The situation is analogous to polynomial interpolation, where fewer points are needed to interpolate a function with a polynomial of higher order, but only with smooth functions that can be effectively approximated by these polynomials. This is not the case of highly irregular and discontinuous functions, for which such approximation is not valid. Furthermore, trying to represent a discontinuous function using high-order regular functions may actually lead to catastrophic artifacts near the discontinuities. Simulating these functions using low order, or even linear functions using small timesteps highly increase the robustness and reduce the errors in such situations.

As the timestep increases, the inaccuracy for large timesteps is degraded with the same order than the one of the method. This imposes a particularly tight control of the suitable timestep for high order methods. For taking advantage of their performance, an efficient adaptive control algorithm is therefore required for tuning the timestep in order to remain within optimal values. The evaluation of the computation error is a good way to control the adequacy of the timestep which is used for the computation. It is possible to embed within the computation of the solution for next step the computation of the possible error interval which provides a way of judging the appropriateness of the timestep size.

Derived from the fourth-order method described above, a convenient way of doing this is to use a derivation of the fifth-order Runge-Kutta algorithm detailed in (Press et al. 1992), modified for computing the error for comparison with an embedded fourth-order evaluation. Using six derivation stages instead of four, we gain an order of accuracy as well as the error evaluation. The timestep control is then carried out by increasing or decreasing the timestep according to the amplitude of the error. Te iteration might even be recomputed with a smaller timestep if the error exceeds a certain threshold. This algorithm was used in the implementations described in (Volino and Magnenat-Thalmann 1997).

Numerical integration, like any other numerical process, is by nature inaccurate. A small and controlled numerical inaccuracy is of no harm to the result, particularly in our case where only the visual aspects are important. However, numerical inaccuracy may produce a more serious side effect: The simulation may become unstable. In such a model, numerical errors accumulate with successive iterations and may diverge, eventually to near-infinite values without any resemblance to physical reality. The model seems to "explode" and there is no hope of recovery.

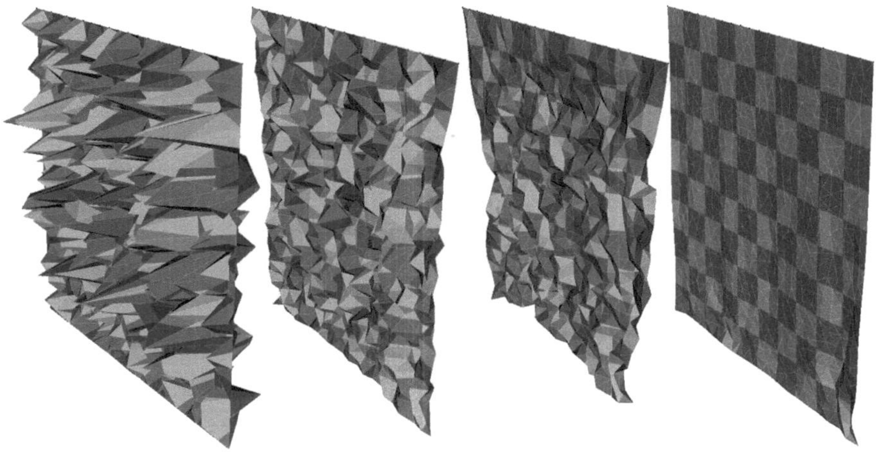

Fig. 3.28 Stability is an essential issue when using explicit numerical integration methods. Stability tests are needed to ensure that the simulation is able to recover from very large deformations (here obtained with large random displacements of vertex positions)

We stated above that accuracy could always be obtained at the expense of computation time. The opposite is unfortunately not always true. While many very simple mechanical models have enough realism for them to be integrated in real-time computation systems, the major limiting factor is not further realism degradation, but numerical instability that is likely to arise.

It is this instability, rather than the numerical inaccuracy itself, which quite often must be controlled in a simulation. The main reason for paying attention to simulation accuracy is not for visual realism, but to prevent the simulation from "exploding" (Fig. 3.28). While small unrealistic artifacts would often go unnoticed in real-time simulation systems, a numeric explosion due to instability systematically leads to unrecoverable effects.

3.3.5.2 Implicit Integration Methods

In order to circumvent the problem of instability, implicit numerical methods are being used. They were first used in the context of cloth simulation by (Baraff et al. 1998).

The most basic implementation of implicit method is the Euler step, which considers finding the future state for which "backward" Euler computation would return the initial state. It performs the computation not using the derivative at the current timestep, but using the predicted derivative for the next timestep. Besides the inverse Euler method, other, more accurate higher-order implicit methods exist, such as the inverse Midpoint method, which remains quite simple but exhibits some instability problems. A simple solution is to interpolate between the equations of the Euler and Midpoint methods, as proposed in (Volino and Magnenat-Thalmann 2005). Higher-order methods, such as the Rosenbrook method, however do not exhibit convincing efficiencies in the field of cloth simulation. Multistep methods, which perform a single-step iteration using a linear combination of several previous states, are other good candidates for a good accuracy-stability compromise. Among them, the second-order Backward Differential Formula (BDF) method has shown some interesting performances, as detailed in (Eberhardt et al. 2000; Hauth et al. 2001; Choi et al. 2002).

Whatever variation is chosen, the major difficulty in using implicit integration methods is that they involve the resolution of a large and sparse linear equation system for each iteration. This being the "frightening" aspect of implicit integration, various approaches have been proposed to resolve this issue.

One of the problems encountered is that the system matrix varies along time, mostly because of the orientation change of the forces between the particles, and also possibly because of the nonlinearities of the mechanical model. In order to optimize the resolution process, one approach is to linearize the problem in order to obtain a matrix which remains constant along the simulation, and constructed once during initialization (Kang et al. 2000). This allows most of the existing numerical resolution libraries to be used. A constant matrix would also allow its inverse to be computed and each iteration then carried out by a simple matrix-vector multiplication, as proposed in (Desbrun et al. 1999). The major problem is that the inverse of a sparse matrix is usually not sparse, and unless drastic approximations the storage difficulty and vector multiplication time severely reduces the interest of this method when the system becomes large. Any-how, when good accuracy and stability are required in the context of nonlinear simulations such as cloth, actual the exact Jacobian corresponding to the current state has to be considered.

Obviously, implicit methods have their advantage in most applications for computer graphics, where numerical stability is the main issue. Most particle systems used for cloth simulation are stiff systems, where the important behavior to be reproduced is the global cloth motion, discarding the unwanted high-frequency phenomena related to particle vibration, which are only the result of the discrete structure. The drawback of implicit methods is that their inaccuracy often translates into numerical damping that degrades the dynamic behavior of animations (Fig. 3.28). While explicit methods require having timesteps adapted to the frequencies of these vibrations to prevent numerical instability, implicit methods can afford dealing with timesteps only adapted to the macroscopic behaviors of the cloth, at the price of poor dynamic accuracy, and also significant per-iteration computation time (Fig. 3.29).

3.3.6 Collision Processing

Virtual objects are determined only by a formal description in the computer's memory. They do not occupy any "real" volume in space. Nothing prevents several such objects from occupying the same volume in virtual space. However, if these objects were to

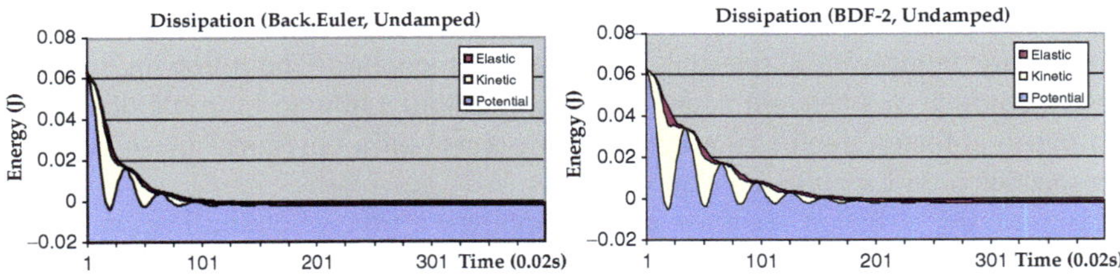

Fig. 3.29 Assessing the accuracy of implicit numerical integration methods can be done by measuring the mechanical energy dissipation caused by numerical errors (here, comparing Implicit Euler and BDF-2 methods for an oscillating square piece of cloth)

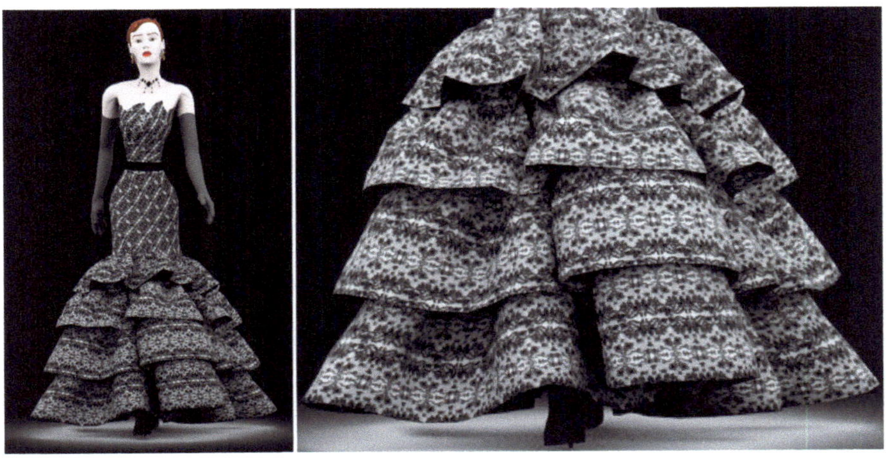

Fig. 3.30 Collision handling is essential for handling virtual garments on bodies, not only for simulating the contact between the cloth and the skin (upper garment part) but also for simulating the contact between different cloth regions (lower garment part)

represent solid objects simultaneously existing in a common scene, they would be unrealistically interpenetrating. Collision management aims to produce, in the virtual world, what is "built in" to the real world: Objects should interact to prevent geometrical interference. The obvious mechanical interactions that occur during contact of real objects have to be completely re-modeled in the computer world (Fig. 3.30).

Collision effects are the consequences of the fact that two objects cannot share the same volume at the same time. When objects touch, interaction forces maintain this volume exclusion. The most important are reaction forces, which oppose geometrical intersection, and then friction forces which prevent objects from sliding against each other. From the point of mechanical simulation, dealing with collisions involves two types of problem:

- *Collision detection*: To find the geometrical contacts between the objects
- *Collision response*: To integrate the resulting reaction and friction effects in the mechanical simulation

These two problems are different in nature: The former is essentially geometrical whereas the latter is more relevant to mechanical modeling. The following sections describe how to manage collision detection efficiently, how to translate this information to collision geometry relevant for response on a polygonal mesh, and the approaches used for collision response.

Before any collision response can be applied, a precise quantification of the geometrical property of the collision has to be computed from the geometrical data carried out by the mesh vertices, as well as the actual involvement of these vertices with respect to basic laws of mechanical momentum conservation.

A good collision response scheme has to exhibit continuity properties: A slight change in the state of the colliding elements should only produce a slight change in the collision response. This property is essential for producing high quality animations where the objects do not "jump" as they slide on each other.

3.3.6.1 Techniques for Collision Detection on Cloth Objects

Detecting object contacts and proximities is, by itself, not very difficult. Depending on the kind of geometrical objects considered, it is always possible to subdivide them into simple primitives. Appropriate mathematical tools are available to determine the geometrical properties of the collisions.

The major difficulty of collision detection is actually related to the number of geometrical primitives that might be implied in collisions. Collision detection would imply testing if every possible couples of potentially colliding primitives do actually collide. Most of the time, a brute-force exploration of all potential couples would lead to a computation time proportional to the square of the number of elements. Thus the real problem is one of complexity. Given a large number of objects of various configurations, the problem concerns how to determine efficiently the collisions between them.

Complexity reduction aims to reduce this quadratic behavior to a smaller function, such as logarithmic or linear. This is done in two ways:

- *The use of tests between pertinent primitive groupings* that might eliminate the need to perform tests between individual elements of these groups. This is usually done by taking advantage of some structural and geometrical consistency between the primitives to be tested.
- *The assumption of structural continuity* of some structural or geometrical properties between successive frames in an animation, allowing incremental computation from frame to frame.

The extraction of relevant geometrical structures from the primitive arrangements to be tested and the consideration of their evolution is the basis of all the optimized algorithms for collision detection. Each of them is adapted to different geometrical contexts, most of them relying on geometrical attributes specific to the context in which they are implemented. Nevertheless, they can be classified into groups depending on the general idea which leads to the complexity reduction. The main groups are:

- *Bounding volumes*, where complex objects or object groups are enclosed within simpler volumes that can be easily tested for collisions. No collision with the volume means no collision with the contained objects to be tested. Most known are bounding boxes, which are defined by the min and max coordinates of the contained objects either in world or in local coordinates (Gottschalk et al. 1996), or bounding spheres (Palmer and Grimsdale 1995; Hubbard 1996), defined by their center and their radius. More advanced are Discrete Orientation Polytopes, bounding polyhedrons defined along arbitrary directions (Klosowsky et al. 1997). Choice of adequate volume is based on how tightly they enclose the objects, how easily they can be geometrically transformed and combined, and how efficiently collision detection is performed between them.
- *Projection methods*, which evaluate possible collisions by considering projections of the scene along several axes or surfaces separately (Cohen et al. 1995). No collision between two projected objects implies no collision between those objects to be tested. A particular application of projection methods involves the 2D rendering of the object using rasterization techniques, most often carried out through high-performance GPU (Heidelberger et al. 2003, 2004).
- *Subdivision methods*, based either on the scene space or on the objects, which decompose the problem into smaller components. They can be space defined, such as voxel methods obtained by subdividing the space with a grid. Objects that do not share a common voxel do not collide. They can also be object regions, usually evaluated through bounding volume techniques. Hierarchical subdivision schemes add efficiency (Held et al. 1995). Space can be defined as octree hierarchies (Fujimura et al. 1983; Yamagushi et al. 1984), whereas objects can be represented as primitive hierarchies, mostly in the form of bounding volume hierarchies (Webb and Gigante 1992; Volino and Magnenat-Thalmann 1994; Van Den Bergen 1997; Mezger et al. 2003; Zachmann and Weller 2006). Collision detection is propagated down in the hierarchy only if the current level presents collision possibility. Most issues involve on efficiently updating the structure as the objects evolve (Larsson and Akenine-Möller 2006; Otaduy et al. 2007).
- *Proximity methods*, which arrange the scene objects according to their geometrical neighborhood, and detect collisions between these objects based on the neighborhood structure. Such structure can be based on minimum distance fields (Fuhrmann et al. 2003), 3D Voronoi domains of the space (Mirtich et al. 1998; Sud et al. 2006) or using Minkowski representations (Gilbert and Foo 1990). Sorting algorithms can also order object in conjunction with projection methods. Collision detection is only performed between neighboring objects. Issues are related on how to update efficiently the structure as the objects evolve.

While most applications use *Discrete Collision Detection* where the objects are checked for collisions at their current locations, *Continuous Collision Detection* takes into account their velocities to pinpoint collision occurrence times precisely (Redon et al. 2002; Hutter and Fuhrmann 2007; Zhang et al. 2007).

All these techniques can be combined in different ways, depending on the various optimizations made possible by the context of the scene. Among possible optimizations, it is possible to take advantage of the consistency of the objects (their size and repartition), and for animations the fact that the scene does not change very much from one frame to another (simple incremental updates made possible by small displacements and constant topologies). Other optimizations include parallel or hardware implementations (Govindaraju et al. 2004). A good overview of collision detection techniques can be found in (Teschner et al. 2005).

3.3.6.2 Collision Response

Collision response intends to enforce the fact that real surfaces cannot cross each other. It may either handle intersections usually by backtracking the motion leading to the surface crossing and integrating the collision effect, and proximities by maintaining a minimum separation distance between the surfaces. In either case, the collision effect is usually applied on the mesh vertices of the colliding elements, which carries the geometrical information of the mesh.

Collision response has to reproduce reaction and friction effects through adequate action in the ongoing mechanical simulation. Its integration in the mechanical simulation system goes through alteration of the mechanical quantities from the value they would have without the collision effects. There are two main ways for handling collision response:

- *Mechanical response*, where the collision reaction is simulated by forces or by force adjustments which reproduce the contact effect
- *Geometrical response*, where the collision reaction is simulated by direct corrections on the positions and velocities of the objects

The mechanical approach is the most formal way of dealing with the problem. The forces or energetic contributions generated from the response can directly be integrated into the mechanical model and simulated. As all the effects are taken into account in the same computation step, the resulting simulation produces an animation where collision response and other mechanical forces add their effects in a compatible way. Reaction is typically modeled by designing a collision penalty force which will repulse the colliding objects from each other and prevent them from intersecting. The repulsion force function is usually designed as a continuous function of the collision distance, and as a piecewise function using simple linear or polynomial intervals. Such approach is for example used in (Lafleur and Magnenat-Thalmann 1991). Designing the optimal shape is difficult, because of all these compromises which depend on the actual mechanical context of the simulation. The biggest issue is to model in a robust way geometrical contact (very small collision distance), in which collision response forces only act in a very small range when considered at the macroscopic scale. This implies the use of very strong and rapidly evolving reaction forces, which are difficult to simulate numerically, since a suitable numerical process should discretize the collision contact duration into timesteps that are numerous enough for an accurate reproduction of the collision effects and which cause problem with the usual simulation timesteps which are usually too large.

The geometrical approach aims to reproduce directly the effects of collision response on the geometrical state of the objects without making use of mechanical forces, and thus in a process separated from the mechanical simulation. It has been extensively used in (Volino and Magnenat-Thalmann 1995–1997). The advantages are obvious: Geometrical constraints are directly enforced by a geometrical algorithm, and the simulation process is relieved from high intensity and highly discontinuous forces or other mechanical parameters, making it faster and more efficient. This drawback however results from this separation: As collision response changes the geometrical state of the objects separately from the mechanical process, nothing ensures the compatibility of this deformation to a correct variation of the mechanical state that would normally result from it. Furthermore, there is no compatible "additivity" of geometrical variations as there is for forces and energy contributions. The resulting collision effects may be incompatible with mechanics, but also between several interacting collisions. All these issues have to be addressed for providing a collision response model that provides acceptable and steady responses between all the frames of an animation.

Collision effects are decomposed into *reaction effects* (normal components), which are the obvious forces preventing the object penetrating into each other, and *friction effects* (tangential components), which model additional forces that oppose the sliding of objects. The most common friction model it the solid Coulombian friction, where friction forces opposing the motion do not exceed reaction forces times a friction coefficient.

3.3.6.3 Repairing Collisions

The complexity of some garments may produce simulations made of numerous cloth surfaces which are involved in complex interactions. Collisions between these surfaces need to be processed accurately using sophisticated algorithms for preventing some intersections, which do not represent a physically consistent state of the cloth.

Most of the time, intersections result from approximate collision detection and response schemes that are not able to enforce consistently the geometrical collision constraints along any situations that may occur during the simulation. Unfortunately, comprehensive methods for ensuring adequate processing of all geometrical collision constraints are complex (detection of numerous mesh collision configurations, interactions between numerous collisions, handling correctly geometrical singularities and numerical errors...) (Bridson et al. 2002). Therefore, they are totally impractical to implement for processing large numbers of collisions with realistic computation times (for example, in the context of simulation of complex garments). It is possible to prevent wrong collision configurations from occurring by tracking their evolution along time (Govindaraju et al. 2005). Meanwhile, faulty initial geometric configurations and nonphysical factors in the simulation context may also lead to surface intersections.

The only way to have a robust simulation system which would safely accommodate any possible collision context in realistic computation times is to design a collision handling system which would not only do its best to process collisions with realistic computation times, but also repair intersections which might have occurred for any reason using dedicated algorithms, to bring the simulation back to a consistent state as quickly as possible. Several untangling algorithms have been designed for this purpose, based on collision contact region identification (Baraff et al. 2003) or intersection contour minimization (Volino and Magnenat-Thalmann 2006).

3.3.7 Real-Time Garment Animation

While simple computation models are able to simulate in real-time the animation of small fabric samples, simulation of virtual garments on animated virtual characters is a very time-consuming process. The biggest performance issues result from the complex and refined meshes necessary to describe the garment geometry in an accurate way. Mechanical simulation of such meshes requires a lot of computational resources to be dedicated to the mechanical evaluations of each mesh elements, along with the numerical integration of the resulting equations. Collision detection furthermore remains an important performance issue despite the use of sophisticated optimization algorithms, the virtual character itself being represented as a very complex geometrical object.

The still huge performance leap necessary for obtaining real-time simulation of complete garments cannot be obtained by further optimization of classic simulation techniques, despite the recent developments on simple models using particle systems, implicit integration and optimized collision detection. They require more drastic simplifications of the simulation process to be carried out, possibly at the expense of mechanical and geometrical accuracy. Among the possibilities are:

- *Geometrical simplification* of the mechanical description of the garment object, using rendering techniques (texturing, bump-mapping, smoothing) for reproducing small details (design features, smooth shapes, folds and wrinkles)
- *Approximations in the collision interactions* between the cloth and the body, for instance using approximate bounding volumes of force fields
- *Low-cost simplified geometric models* for animating the cloth object, which approximate the mechanical behavior and motion of the cloth into predefined geometric deformations. Problems involve the design of adequate predefined motions that would represent the properties of the cloth in the many different mechanical contexts garments could be involved. These motions are usually defined using analytic functions adapted to a particular context, or by automatic processes such as neural networks "learning" the cloth behavior from actual simulations (Grzezczuk et al. 1998; Cordier and Magnenat-Thalmann 2005)

- *Hybrid context-sensitive simulation frameworks* which simplify the computation according to the current interaction context of garment regions, possibly mixing together rough mechanical simulation with small-scale specific simulation of features such as wrinkles (Kang et al. 2000)
- *Integrated body-and-garment simulations* where the cloth is defined directly as a processing of the skin, either as texture and bump-mapping (suitable for stretch cloth) or using local deformations reacting to the body motion using simplified mechanics (Cordier et al. 2002)

All these techniques can be combined for designing a real-time system for garment animation, provided that the body animation system and the rendering pipeline is efficient enough so support these features with adequate frame rate.

3.3.7.1 Real-Time Garment Animation on a Virtual Character

In this section, we intend to demonstrate the process of integrating the simulation of garments on an animated character in real-time. The main idea of this process is to create a unified representation of the body and the garment in a single object, by extrapolating the skinning information from the body surface to the garment surface. This extrapolated information would then be used either for animating the garment geometrically (through the same skinning deformation as the one used for animating the body), either to give to the mechanical simulator information for simplified collision detection between the cloth and the local body surfaces.

The automatic skinning extrapolation tracks the relevant features of the body shape ruling the animation of any vertex of the garment surface. This algorithm can be designed by extending a proximity map (nearest mesh feature algorithm) with additional visibility considerations for pinpointing the actual geometrical dependencies between the surfaces of the body and the cloth. A smooth blending between the weights of several nearest points smoothes the transitions between body parts (Fig. 3.31). Additional smoothness criteria can also be also embedded so as to prevent any jaggy deformation over the garment surface. Further optimizations, such as the reduction of bone dependency count, should also be performed for reducing the computational time of skinning animation.

Collision data is obtained from the same nearest-feature algorithm used in the skinning extrapolation scheme, and optimized with specific distance and visibility considerations. Hence, for each vertex of the garment mesh, a set of vectors relating the nearest body features is stored (Fig. 3.32). Then, during the animation, these vectors are skinned using the corresponding vertex weights, and collision distance and orientation can then be extracted from these vectors for adequate collision processing.

The mechanical engine is a fast and optimized implementation of the tensile cloth model described in Section 3.3.4. It is associated to an implicit Backward-Euler integration scheme, which offers good performance along adequate robustness

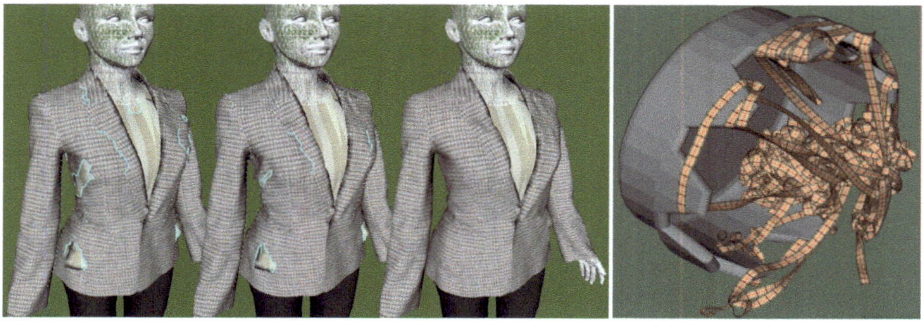

Fig. 3.31 A robust cloth simulation system should not only process collisions properly, but also "repair" any intersecting surfaces, on complex garment involving several layers of cloth (*left*) as well as on more challenging situations too complex for being handled comprehensively (*right*)

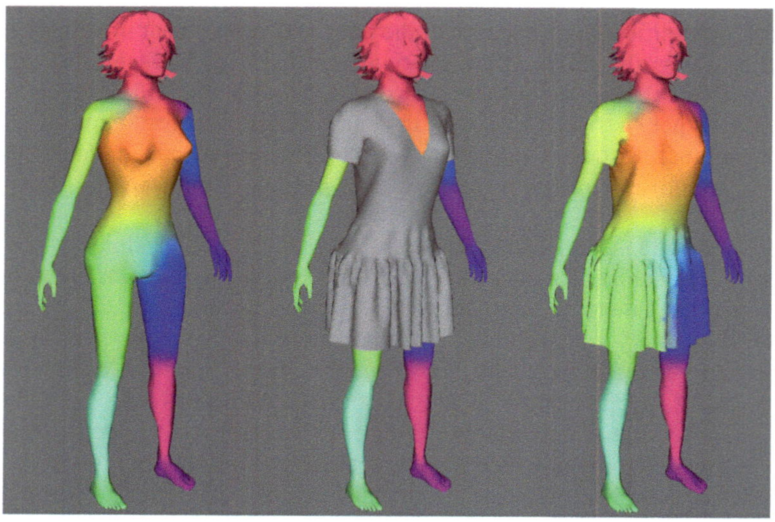

Fig. 3.32 The skinning weights of the mesh element (shown by the *bone colors*) (*left*) are extrapolated on the garment surface (*right*) using through a smooth blending of the weights of the nearest mesh features

in this simulation context. Through the use of an accurate mechanical model that offers good representation of the mechanical properties of cloth, it is possible to obtain a fairly realistic simulation which can suit the needs of fast fitting preview, during body motion, as well as body or garment resizing (Figs. 3.33 and 3.34).

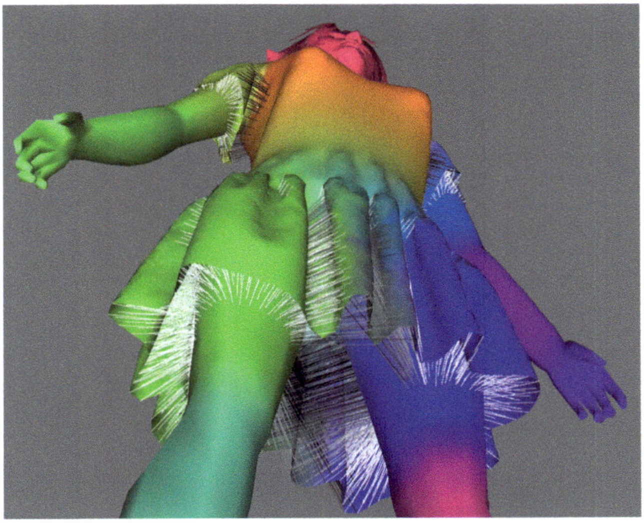

Fig. 3.33 Collision information is stored as vectors relating the orientation and distance of the potentially colliding body surfaces. These vectors are deformed by the skinning process during the body animation

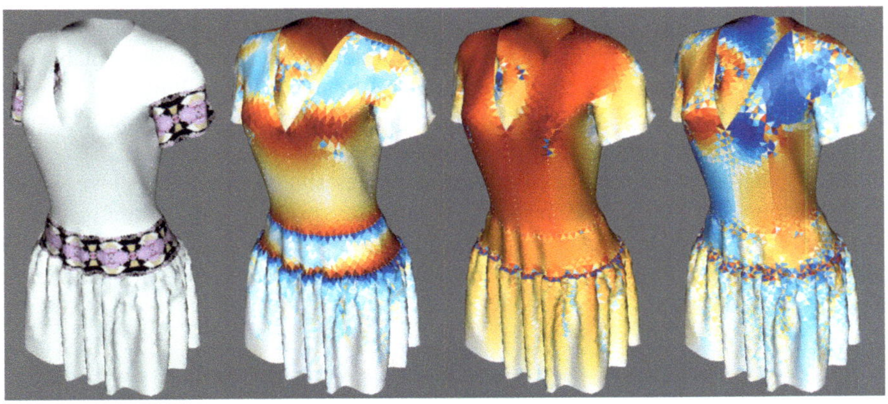

Fig. 3.34 Extraction of the weft, warp and shear tensile deformation values on the cloth surface using the 2D fabric surface coordinates of the patterns and the initial 3D shape of garment

3.4 Touching Virtual Textiles

While cloth animation and rendering techniques have dramatically improved during the last 2 decades (see Section 3.3.1), the *interaction modalities* with cloth-like deformable surfaces have not followed this evolution. Handling virtual textiles traditionally requires the use of a mouse and a keyboard. But humans are used to

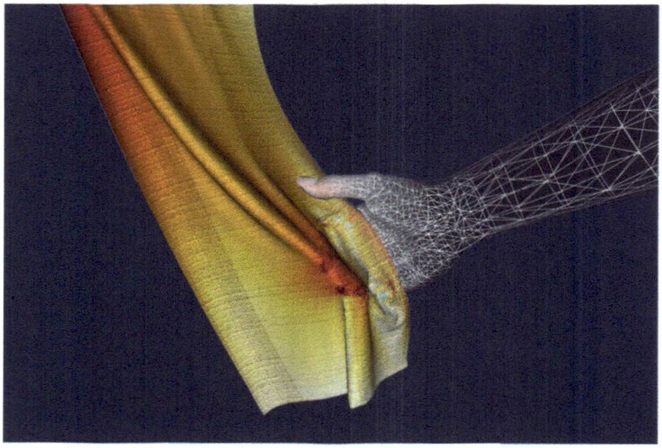

Fig. 3.35 Touching virtual textiles: dream or reality?

skin contact with clothing materials and instinctively strongly rely on their feeling of touch when handling textiles. Providing the sensation of touching virtual textiles in the context of three-dimensional computer simulation environments can, therefore, significantly increase the realism and believability of the user experience. This kind of enhanced interaction is made possible by *haptic devices*, novel interfaces capable of mediating the sensation of touch. Haptic interaction with deformable 3D textiles can speed up the process of handling and creating digital clothes. Moreover, it allows to assess the specific surface and material properties of 3D objects representing real products (e.g. during the online purchase of real garments).

Ideally, an interface for touching virtual clothes should provide a glove which would display the user's hand in the 3D simulation space (as shown by Fig. 3.35), and return all associated feedback according to the specific textile material and performed actions. But how far is it possible to provide the sensation of touching virtual textiles?

3.4.1 Haptic Interaction with Virtual Textiles: The Problems to Solve

A multimodal virtual reality experience which allows touching simulated textiles implies the progress of a number of specific technologies beyond the current state of the art. Their successful development and integration requires the solution of several research problems ranging from the conceptual design of the desired system functionalities to the evaluation and validation of the realized software/hardware components.

3.4.1.1 Abstraction of the Real World Scenario

Most everyday interactions are something self-understood and obvious. Especially touching clothes belongs to the most natural everyday activities which are performed several times a day, whenever handling garments (dressing, undressing, straightening, adjusting, folding, etc.). However, trying to reproduce these so obvious actions in a virtual reality context requires an in-depth knowledge of the human sense of touch, and a solid understanding of how the physical attributes of textile materials are sensed and interpreted.

In order to stimulate the sense of touch through digital cues, researchers need to abstract the real world scenario and decompose the action of touching clothes into a set of simplified processes which can be reproduced by VR technology:

- How do humans perceive objects? What are the peculiarities of the tactile and the kinesthetic senses? What is the "sensing resolution" of the human hands, and what are the perceptual mechanisms which allow our touch receptors to handle tactile and kinesthetic stimuli?
- Which physical properties are really relevant when perceiving textiles from a visual and a haptic viewpoint?
- What are adequate methods for objectively measuring the relevant physical properties on real fabrics?

3.4.1.2 Development of Physically Based Simulation Techniques to Render the Cloth Behavior According to the Specified Fabric Parameters

Once the requirements of a VR application for handling digital clothes are identified, the challenge is to define an encoding/decoding strategy to transform real physical attributes into digital touch signals. This correlation must be perfectly consistent with the performed action.

From the haptic viewpoint, sensing and reproducing *both* tactile and force sensations is essential in order to fully exploit the sense of touch. At the same time, these multiple stimuli affect the textiles' visual behavior, which reacts to the user's touch. This intricate interrelation requires physical models capable of considering various inputs from the different perceptual modalities. Multimodal VR simulation is based on software modules tackling these main problems:

- What is the best tactile rendering strategy which provides appropriate stimuli to the fingertip skin according to the fabric surface patterns?
- How to compute the force-feedback to the user according to the performed interaction and the specific kinesthetic behavior of the fabric sample?
- How to efficiently design and implement a visual display model that enables realistic rendering of the textile in real time?

3.4.1.3 Design and Realization of a Haptic Interface Able to Provide Both Tactile and Kinesthetic Stimuli

Handling multimodal interaction with virtual textiles requires, next to specialized software, also adequate hardware components capable of transforming the computed signals into tangible physical stimuli which can be perceived by the user. Due to its innovative character, haptic interaction with virtual clothes requires a dedicated solution to several non-trivial technological problems which have not been tackled by commercial devices yet. In particular, this concerns finding solutions for achieving efficient multisensory integration and synchronization. In this endeavor, following research questions are of fundamental relevance:

- How to integrate a force-feedback device with tactile arrays avoiding that the two components interfere with each other?
- What is the best strategy to synchronize the multiple sensory feedbacks to create a consistent and plausible experience?

3.4.1.4 Cross-Modal Validation of the Complete System

The final working system requires a thorough validation proving its operational reliability and realism. Several experiments need to be performed in order to assess if the VR system works in the predicted way and if the user is able to operate it as expected. While using a virtual reality system necessarily involves initial learning, the effort required to acquire the new skill of touching virtual textiles should be comparable to using new interaction technology devices without introducing additional complexity. Concrete evaluation issues which should be addressed include:

- How far does the interaction in virtual reality match the real experience at different perception modalities?
- What are the effects of excluding selected perceptual modalities, and how does this affect the system usability?

Even though specifically addressing the multimodal simulation of textiles, the challenges described above represent a scientific roadmap which can be universally followed when tackling the visual and haptic simulation of any deformable object.

3.4.2 The Sense of Touch

The exact perceptual mechanisms of the human sense of touch are not yet well understood. Understanding the haptic sense in humans is a fundamental requirement for reproducing the sensation of touch. But the complex relationships between stimulus, perception and interpretation are largely unexplored. Psychophysical studies of the mechanisms underlying haptic perception can provide important insight e.g. in the sensing resolution of different mechanoreceptors and proprioceptors. In this context, a reliable neurobiological classification of touch receptors in the skin can provide insightful information about the way edges, surfaces and volumes are perceived, and can serve as a basis for reproducing digital touch sensations.

The human perception of touch can be divided into the tactile and kinesthetic sensing modalities. These modalities respectively deal with the perception and interpretation of surface properties and of the movements associated with haptic exploration strategies.

3.4.2.1 The Tactile Sense

The *tactile sense* relies on sensory nerves and receptors which have their highest density on the fingertips. The thousands of individual nerve fibers below the skin of the human hand are populated by four principal classes of mechanoreceptors responding to skin deformation such as pressure, stretch and vibration (Rowe et al. 2006). Receptors fall into two broad groups responding to static and dynamic skin deformation respectively.

The first group is responsive to *static* mechanical displacement of skin tissues and concerns slowly adapting (SA) receptors and afferent fibers. Its two classes innervate Merkel disks (SA-I) and Ruffini organs (SA-II). Merkel disks are selectively sensitive to edges, corners, and curvatures (Johnson 2001). Ruffini organs are sensitive to static skin stretch and perceive hand shape and finger position through the stretch patterns on the skin.

The afferents of the second group are insensitive to static skin deformation, but display a high *dynamic* sensitivity instead. These dynamic receptors fall into two principal classes. The Meissner corpuscles are rapidly adapting (RA) receptors responsible for detecting slip between the skin and an object held in the hand (Johnson et al. 2000). The Pacinian Corpuscles (PC) are highly sensitive receptors which respond to distant events, e.g. vibrations mediated through a tool.

3.4.2.2 The Kinesthetic Sense

The *kinesthetic sense* is mediated by proprioceptive sensors which provide information about spatial localization and determine human awareness to the body movements. Receptors populate muscle spindles, Golgi tendon organs, as well as in and around joints (Proske 2006). Muscle spindles are found in skeletal muscles and provide information on muscle length and rate of muscular contraction. They consist of intrafusal muscles fibers innervated by gamma motor neurons, and are important in maintaining muscle tone. Golgi tendon organs are located at the junction of a tendon and a muscle; their function is to sense muscle contraction force. Joint kinesthetic receptors are found within and around the joint capsule and are responsible for sensing joint position and movement.

3.4.3 Rendering Touch Signals

Generating digital signals aiming at the stimulation of the sense of touch in a virtual reality context requires knowing the nature of these signals in the real situation. But how does the process of evaluating the physical consistency of real objects occur? How do humans e.g. evaluate the make and the quality of real textiles? In the textile industry, where this question is of particular importance, the sum of the sensations experienced when a fabric is touched or manipulated with the fingers is commonly defined as "fabric hand" (see Section 3.3.2). Handling textiles in a virtual reality context requires returning to the final user precisely those stimuli which can be considered more relevant for assessing fabric hand. This includes delivering the appropriate haptic signals directed to the tactile and kinesthetic senses, while appropriately matching the visual cues. The computation of these stimuli is called *haptic rendering*, and can be divided into tactile and force rendering.

3.4.3.1 The Haptic Interaction Process

Figure 3.36 shows a typical haptic interaction process describing the usage of a force-feedback device. The user of a haptic system typically operates a haptic interface through an end effector (1) and perceives contact forces through the skin surface (2) by both the tactile and the kinesthetic senses. These haptic stimuli are interpreted in the brain (3), which in turn decides the further exploration strategy and the movements to perform (4) for the interaction with the virtual object. The user

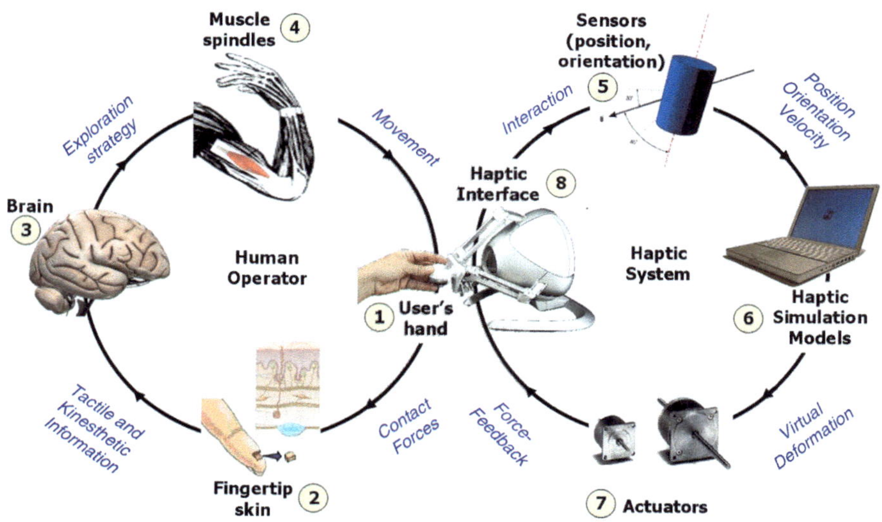

Fig. 3.36 Haptic interaction process: there is a reciprocal dependency of the dual loop concerning the human operator and the haptic system. In the middle: a Novint Falcon (Courtesy of Novint, Inc.)

operates the haptic device and the resulting motion is sensed (5) by the device's position and orientation trackers. The tracked input data (such as fingertip position and speed) is used to compute the deformations of the virtual model of the touched object (6) according to the user's actions. The forces arising on the touched object due to the computed deformations are then transmitted to the haptic interface, which through its actuators (7) returns a force-feedback to the user (8) reflecting the state change of the virtual object.

Even though the haptic interface displayed in the figure is a force-feedback device, the described haptic interaction process also applies for tactile and combined tactile-kinesthetic interaction.

But what is the best way to generate haptic signals, and is it possible to evaluate their efficiency in terms of realism and believability? Solutions for the rendering of appropriate tactile and force cues reproducing the sensation of stroking virtual objects are still largely unexplored. In order to evaluate the realism and believability of haptic simulations, psychophysical studies compare the quantitative values used in the simulation (acquired from objective measurements) to what is subjectively felt by the end user of the system. This is done both in the real and in the virtual scenario, as well as for different perceptual modalities, since the efficient synchronization of realistic tactile, kinesthetic and visual stimuli is a highly complex problem which requires coping with different data models and high computational costs.

3.4.3.2 Tactile Rendering

One of the main problems in the domain of tactile rendering is the definition of appropriate skin excitation patterns, whose nature and origin are not well understood even in real situations. Their simulation in a virtual environment context needs, therefore, solutions for relating the complex mechanical properties of the object's surface to the local topology of the fingertip's skin. Moreover, many aspects of the exploratory movement (such as speed, contact pressure and direction) strongly influence tactile sensing and must be accurately taken into account. Early attempts to encode tactile perception of fabrics (Govindaraj et al. 2003) took advantage of surface measurements performed with the Kawabata System (see Section 3.3.2), whose probe and instrumentation accurately correlate the measured quantities with subjective assessment of the textile surface. These measurements, therefore, return the *perceived* textile surface, since they provide an approximation of the surface after it has been filtered through the surface/skin interface. In order to use the measured parameters for generating appropriate tactile stimuli to the users' skin, tactile rendering of 3D deformable surfaces such as textiles requires defining three main layers (Summers et al. 2005).

1. A surface model, describing physical and geometrical properties
2. A localization layer, mapping the fingertip's position to the surface model and sending tactile cues to a tactile renderer
3. A tactile renderer, converting filtered tactile stimuli into signals for the tactile array hardware

In the particular case of tactile manipulation of virtual 3D fabrics, the mechanical input to the skin's mechanoreceptors can be approximated from KES-f *roughness and friction profiles* of textile samples. This data can be used to generate driving signals for the tactile stimulator array. A spatial-frequency spectrum is computed considering the movement direction and the surface model. Taking into account the speed of the movement, the spatial frequency spectrum is converted into temporal-frequency components. By application of appropriate band pass filter functions, the temporal-frequency spectrum is reduced to match only two amplitudes which are then weighted according to the surface model, generating a 40-Hz and a 320-Hz channel (Allerkamp et al. 2007). Virtual objects encountered during an active exploration of the workspace by the user are converted into appropriate patterns of tactile stimulation using this strategy and rendered on the fingertips through tactile actuators capable of generating tactile stimuli.

3.4.3.3 Force Rendering

KES-f measurements can provide useful information for quantifying the forces acting on cloth materials. These parameters are used by physical simulation models to animate the textile according to the user interaction. Force rendering modules compute the forces arising during the interaction and send them to the haptic hardware for delivering the appropriate force-feedback. In order to optimize the efficiency of the computations, the cloth model is structured into two areas: (1) the whole fabric specimen influenced by the interaction (global shape) and (2) the contact region directly around the fingertip touching the fabric (local geometry).

The fabric's *global shape* is described by a real-time textile simulation model (see Section 3.3.3). The global simulation is optimized for robustness and is capable of displaying in real time the anisotropic large-scale behavior of the whole fabric at a centimeter-size resolution, taking into account global physical parameters.

The *local geometry* reflects the immediate surface changes arising at the contact points and calculates the interaction forces between the virtual fabric and the virtual finger. This layer must directly feed the haptic device through a force renderer approximating forces arising from local deformations. Moreover, it should efficiently interpolate this local behavior with the global motion through a reciprocal synchronization. Figure 3.37 displays a piece of textile showing local and global areas.

The deformations of the local geometry arising from haptic interaction occur within a time frame of milliseconds, which is small enough to be described sufficiently well by the laws of elasticity, neglecting external forces (e.g. gravity). Therefore, deformations of the local geometry can be described by a simple linear mass-spring model without a significant loss of accuracy (Böttcher et al. 2007). Such a mass-spring system can describe the textile deformation forces by looking at changes in warp and weft directions for each triangular element of the mesh. The forces are then integrated over the triangle and distributed among the particles. To provide a comprehensive modeling of the forces acting in the contact region, the local geometry model should take into consideration:

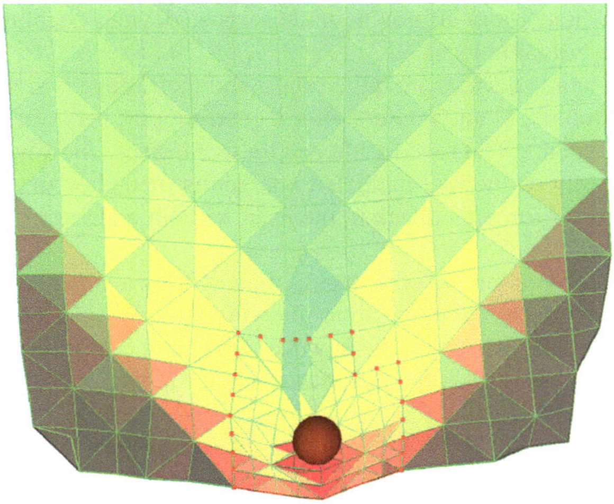

Fig. 3.37 Simulated textile displaying the global polygon mesh and the local geometry around the contact area

- *Tensile forces* measured by the elongation in warp and weft direction compared to the rest state under the assumption that the stretch is constant over a triangle
- *Shearing forces* generated by a movement parallel to a fixed axis, taking the KES-f measurements as a reference
- *Bending forces* computed proportionally to the angle between two neighboring triangles. Folds are displayed only over the edges of the triangles. In contrast to shearing and tensile forces, bending forces are not evenly distributed throughout the triangle
- *Damping forces* modeling the energy dissipation during the deformation and ensuring simulation stability. These damping forces are opposing forces counteracting the stretch, shear and bend motions independently from each other

Efficient and accurate force rendering methods can only be useful in combination with appropriate haptic interfaces, capable of returning the computed forces to the human operator.

3.4.4 Haptic Interfaces

The lack of detailed knowledge of the functioning of the human perceptual system and the difficulties encountered when digitally encoding/decoding touch signals surely represent non-trivial challenges which still need to be satisfactorily solved. But there are also other factors which preclude the application development in the domain of computer haptics. One of the main obstacles to the widespread adoption of complex touch-enabled VR systems is currently represented by the limited availability of efficient-and-affordable multipurpose devices enabling direct haptic interaction with virtual objects.

Commercial haptic devices are quite robust and their usage is simplified by a set of developing toolkits. Manufacturers offer a good support network and continuous product improvements. The functionality of these interfaces, however, is somewhat limited, as they rely on the tool-mediated interaction metaphor and mostly provide a single point-based force-feedback to the user, without addressing distributed tactile feedback.

Research prototypes, on the other hand, often address a larger variety of interaction modalities while at the same time allowing experimental research on more specific problems. Their drawback, however, lies in the high costs and delicate hardware handling, as well as the lack of technical support.

3.4.4.1 Commercial Devices

Among the most well-known commercially available haptic devices figure the SensAble Phantom, the ForceDimension omega, as well as the more recent Novint Falcon. The first two are multi-purpose high-precision devices for haptic-based applications in research and industry, while the latter is designed as a game controller providing force-feedback in entertainment applications.

The SensAble Phantom and ForceDimension omega product lines display different models to meet varying requirements in terms of workspace, force and space resolution, and degrees of freedom. Novint's Falcon is announced to be the first of a new category of touch products for the consumer market aiming at replacing the mouse or joystick. The figures below show a SensAble PHANTOM® Desktop™ haptic device (left) and a Novint Falcon (right) (Figs. 3.38 and 3.39).

3.4.4.2 Tactile Actuators

Actuators delivering distributed tactile feedback are currently only available as research prototypes. During the last decade, different approaches have been used to provide tactile cues describing the surface texture of the virtual object and the contact between object and skin. A variety of electromechanical drive mechanisms with different specifications of contactor spacing, working bandwidth and output amplitude have been developed. They either apply tangential forces through piezoelectric-bimorph actuators or normal forces to the skin through moving-coil technology or shape memory alloy (Magnenat-Thalmann et al. 2007a). In most cases, the intention is not to reconstruct the small-scale surface topology of the object in terms of a virtual surface. Instead, the goal is to reproduce the *perceptual consequences* of the surface topology. This can be achieved through the delivery of appropriate excitation patterns at different frequencies (e.g. one 40-Hz and one 320-Hz channel) to stimulate the various populations of touch receptors in the skin.

The tactile component shown in Fig. 3.40 uses piezoelectric bimorphs to drive 24 contactors in a 6×4 array on the fingertip, with a spacing of 2 mm between

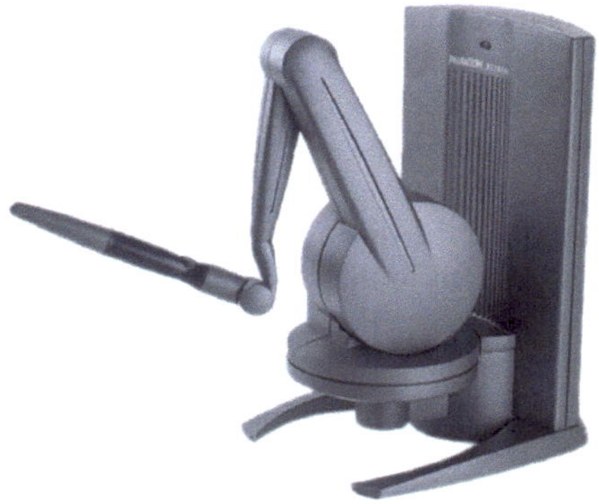

Fig. 3.38 SensAble PHANTOM® Desktop™ haptic device. © SensAble Technologies, Inc. PHANTOM, PHANTOM Desktop, SensAble, and SensAble Technologies, Inc. are trademarks or registered trademarks of SensAble Technologies, Inc.

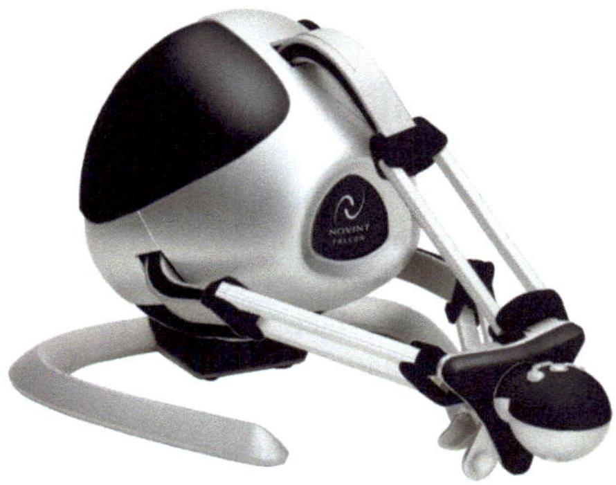

Fig. 3.39 Novint Falcon haptic device (black version). © Novint Technologies, Inc. Falcon, Novint, and Novint Technologies, Inc. are either the trademarks or the registered trademarks of Novint

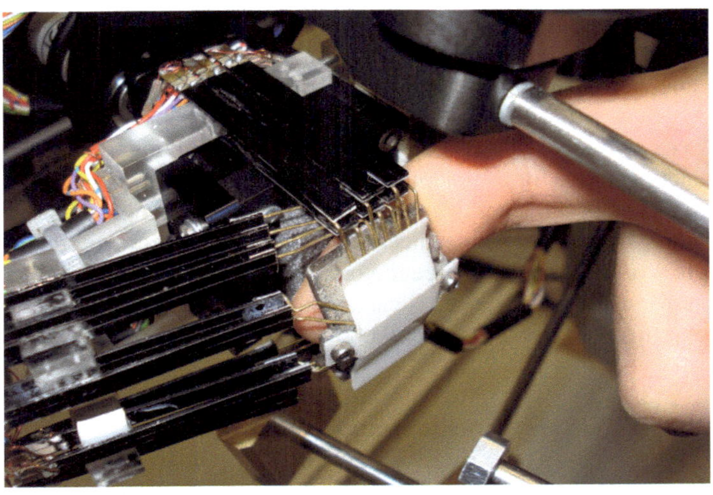

Fig. 3.40 Piezoelectric tactile array

contactor centers. It represents an improved version of the array described in (Summers et al. 2005) with the drive mechanism placed to the side and ahead of the finger, rather than below the contactor surface. With one such array on the index finger and one on the thumb, this positioning of the drive mechanism allows the finger to move close to the thumb so that a virtual textile can be manipulated between the tips of the finger and the thumb. The corresponding tactile stimuli are transferred to the skin during active manipulation.

While tactile actuators are capable of describing the surface roughness and friction on the virtual textile surface, they do not provide any information concerning the global shape of the textile sample, its weight or the tensile/bending forces acting on it. This dynamic behavior, calculated by force rendering software modules, is rendered by the associated force-feedback device. Providing the force sensation on different spots of the hand simultaneously requires a multipoint force-feedback device.

3.4.4.3 Multipoint Force-Feedback Devices

While the most commercially available haptic devices return a force-feedback on one single point (in some cases on two) through a stylus-like probe, the most intuitive force-feedback device for directly manipulating thin objects is most probably a glove-like interface. In order to be able to reproduce the forces arising during textile manipulation, such a device must be expressly conceived for the accurate generation of light forces.

Among the different types of touch-gloves, hand-exoskeletons are capable of efficiently delivering precise forces. They are mainly divided into two categories: *multi-phalanx devices* generate forces along each finger's phalanx in a fixed direction, while *fingertip devices* can generate forces only on the fingertips, but in any arbitrary direction in 3D space. As the second type of functionality promises the best results for assessing thin objects in 3D space, researchers have realized an actuated and sensorised hand exoskeleton in form of a fingertip device (Fontana et al. 2007), depicted in Fig. 3.41.

The device is composed by two actuated and sensorised finger exoskeletons (one for the index and one for the thumb) and is body-grounded. It is connected to a sensorised mechanical tracker that provides the absolute position and orientation of the operator's hand. The whole mechanism has four degrees of freedom, even though it is actuated with only three motors, thanks to the coupling of the last joint with the previous one. The device is capable of exerting a continuous force of 5 N on the fingertips with a resolution of 0.005 N.

3.4.4.4 Integration and Synchronization

In order to provide a unified haptic interface delivering a comprehensive feeling of interacting with virtual textiles, tactile actuators and force-feedback devices must

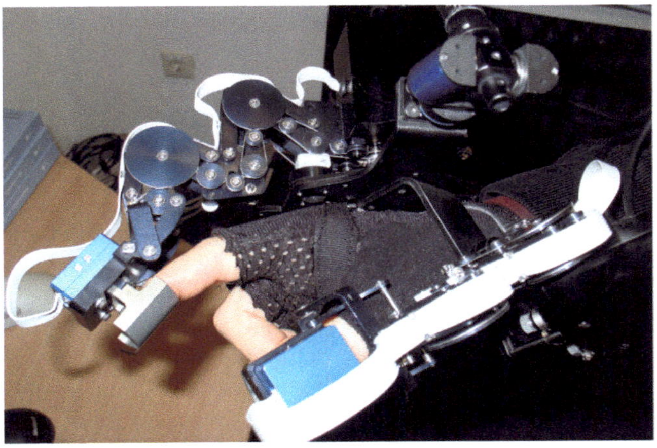

Fig. 3.41 A hand-exoskeleton for manipulating light objects

be integrated into one single interface. Similarly, different simulation modules calculating visual, tactile and force-feedback must be efficiently synchronized in order to ensure a consistent and physically plausible experience.

The hardware integration of the force-feedback device with the tactile actuators should ensure the delivery of the mechanical stimulations to the fingertip without interferences between the devices. Two main problems should be avoided. Firstly, the global forces conveyed by the force-feedback device should not load the pins of the tactile array. Secondly, the mass of the tactile array drive mechanism should not load the force sensor. A possible solution is to attach the drive mechanism of the tactile actuators directly to the final link of the force-feedback device. The tactile pins vibrate then through holes in the force plate attached to the force sensor's load flange (Fontana et al. 2007).

The simulation synchronization is necessary at runtime in order to ensure that different perceptual stimuli correspond with the user interaction. This is particularly the case around the contact area between virtual textile and finger, as it represents the main center of interest during fabric handling. The tactile feedback is computed according to a localization function, which maps the fingertip's position to the surface model and sends tactile cues to the tactile rendering unit. Visual and tactile consistency is ensured by matching the tactile surface model to the fabric's texture used for graphical rendering. Visual and kinesthetic consistency is ensured through the global/local simulation mechanism. Kinesthetic instabilities between the global and local shapes at the contour of the contact area can be avoided by assuming constant velocity at the border of the local geometry and by removing additional forces from the corresponding particles. The visual transition between the global and the local mesh representations is ensured by smoothing the textile's contours and edges through an appropriate mesh subdivision scheme. This can be applied on-the-fly to the mesh at rendering time, and allows subdividing each geometric polygon into several pieces fitting adequately the local surface curvature, increasing the geometric rendering quality.

3.4.5 The EU Project HAPTEX: Concepts and Solutions

The European Research Project HAPTEX – HAPtic Sensing of Virtual TEXtiles – successfully developed a multimodal virtual reality system capable of rendering the sensation of stroking and manipulating a piece of three-dimensional digital fabric (Magnenat-Thalmann et al. 2007a). The resulting simulation system uses physical models based on real measurements to define the visual, tactile and kinesthetic representation of the virtual textile. The sense of touching virtual textiles is provided by a new generation haptic interface integrating kinesthetic and tactile actuators. The HAPTEX System allows its user to select a fabric material and interact with a specimen, as Fig. 3.42 shows, feeling a combined force and tactile feedback.

3.4.5.1 Validation

The evaluation of the HAPTEX system assessed all different aspects of the simulation. The results of the physical simulation framework reproducing the virtual fabric

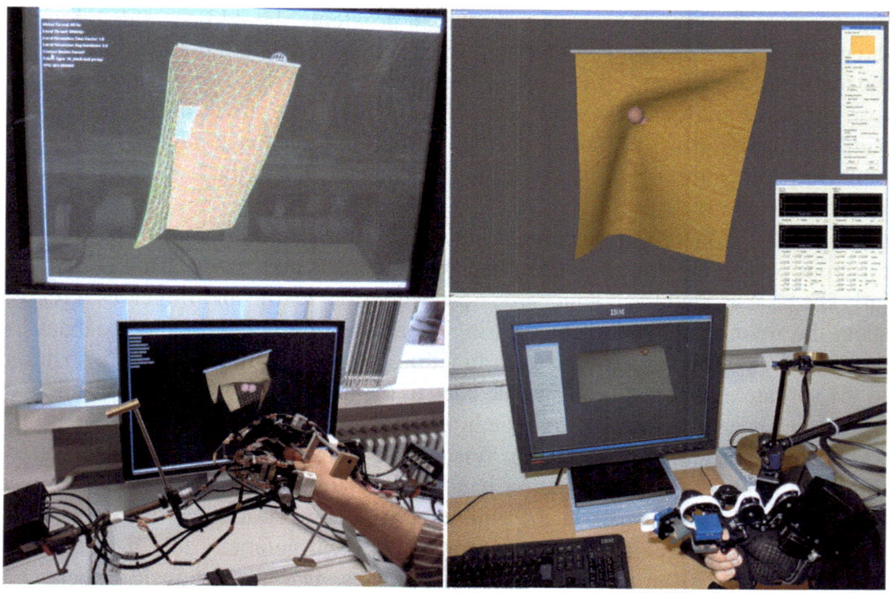

Fig. 3.42 The HAPTEX real-time textile simulation framework (*top*) and the final HAPTEX system in two different configurations (early version *bottom left*, final system *bottom right*) (HAPTEX Consortium 2008a)

were compared with the motion of real fabrics. Likewise, all different system components were validated separately. Finally, the complete system was assessed in terms of functionality, comparing the results from a subjective evaluation of real fabrics and a subjective evaluation of virtual fabrics. Cross-modal interactions were analyzed through experiments carried out in two variants: with and without vision.

The physical and visual realism of the virtual textile simulation was assessed through three different evaluation methods, which were performed on a variety of textile samples (as Fig. 3.43 shows): static simulation of fabric drape (top left), dynamic simulation of fabric falling down from a fixed stand (bottom left), and dynamic simulation of fabric on a moving sphere (top right).

The final system evaluation required to manipulate virtual textiles and rate the properties felt during interaction. These ratings were compared to those obtained in an equivalent assessment of the real textiles, and to physical data obtained using the Kawabata measurement system and other techniques. Assessed properties included tensile stiffness, surface roughness/friction, and bending stiffness/weight/drapeability. An evaluation procedure was defined and followed under different operating conditions (tests were performed in "full vision" or "wireframe" mode, as shown in Fig. 3.43, bottom right). For the complex case of evaluating bending stiffness (difficult to assess due to the low forces arising during such interactions), the evaluator was asked to make a visual assessment. The performed evaluations

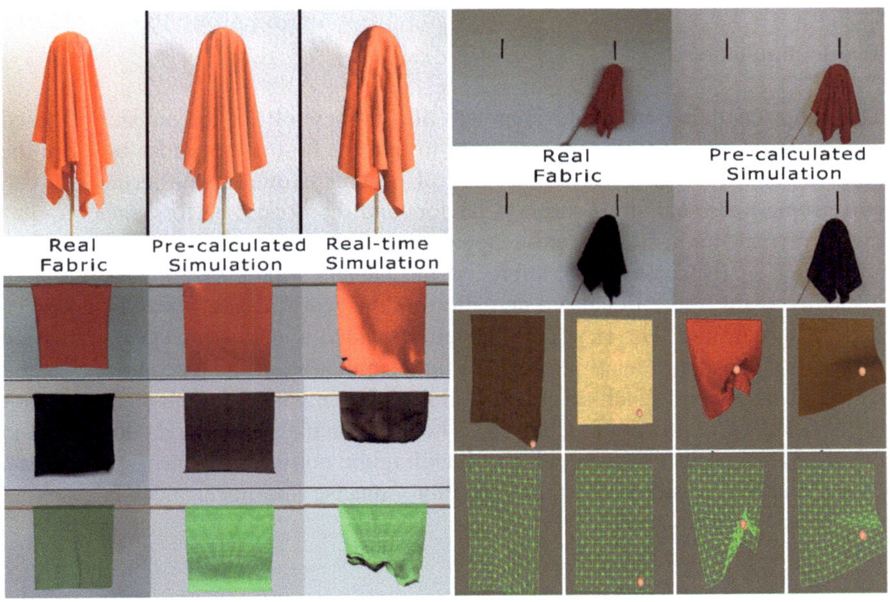

Fig. 3.43 Different validation tests: static simulation of fabric drape (*top left*), dynamic simulation of fabric falling down from a fixed stand (*bottom left*), and dynamic simulation of fabric on a moving sphere (*top right*). On the bottom right, manipulation procedures for assessing different physical properties

provided a good correspondence between the ratings of the virtual textiles and the real textiles especially for the properties of tensile stiffness, surface roughness and surface friction (HAPTEX Consortium 2008b).

3.4.5.2 Results

Considering the state of art in the field of haptics, computer graphics and human perception at the beginning of the project, it is unquestionable that the HAPTEX project posed several very demanding challenges in both the technical area and the scientific domain. The challenge is even stronger if the resource and time constraints of the project are taken into account. However, the HAPTEX system successfully achieved its goal to offer a sophisticated virtual environment for the manipulation of virtual textiles. A range of technical advancements was achieved in order to produce the system, including the implementation of an efficient virtual textile model derived from measurements on real textiles (allowing real-time interaction and offering a significantly more realistic experience than existing simulations of deformable objects), and the implementation of touch stimulation with variable spatial distribution over the skin (combining, for the first time, distributed tactile stimulation with force-feedback, using a tactile rendering strategy which is designed to reproduce the sensation of a real surface).

Textile Simulation

The major challenge in the development of a framework for the physically based simulation of virtual textiles is generally to find the best compromise between the high requirements in terms of mechanical accuracy (quantitative accuracy with anisotropic nonlinear strain-stress behavior) and the drastic performance requirements of real-time and interactive applications. The main limitation of previous simulation systems consists in imprecise mechanical simulation models, the main difficulty being the efficient computation of the realistic non-linear behavior of fabrics in real time. The HAPTEX System provided a unique physical simulation framework capable of handling the real-time simulation of the piece of textile and its visualization, and synchronizing this global motion with the small-scale behavior of fabrics driving the haptic feedback. The new calculation methods developed in the HAPTEX project were capable of handling the non-linear behavior of textiles, even for real time simulations. But therefore, precise non-linear mechanical input parameters were required.

Fabric Measurements

Physical properties of real fabrics were provided by the database of fabric parameters realized in the context of HAPTEX. The database covered a wide range of textile parameters, including nonlinear elasticity properties, obtained from specific fabric measurements (see Section 3.3.2).

The specifications of the HAPTEX Project required several modifications to the originally planned standard test procedures, which resulted in significant advancements with respect to the state of the art in textile measurements. Among others, traditional tensile testing was improved developing the new "step-tensile" test method. Moreover, the output of KES-F measurements was digitized and filtered in order to optimize the measured signals.

Force-Feedback and Tactile Rendering

A main limit of existing approaches for the haptic rendering of deformable objects is the discrepancy between the real-time needs of the haptic device with an update rate of 1,000 Hz and the high computational costs of the objects simulation resulting in a much lower update rate. The haptic rendering framework of HAPTEX proved to be capable of bridging the different update rates. The part of the deformable object in contact with the user was simulated by an intermediate layer. While this solution was specifically designed for dealing with the interaction with virtual fabrics, it offers further development potential for being applied to a larger class of deformable objects. Moreover, unlike many other haptic rendering systems, the HAPTEX force renderer allowed handling two simultaneous contact interactions, namely with the user's thumb and index finger.

Little research was previously done in the domain of tactile rendering of virtual textiles. The HAPTEX consortium was among the first groups investigating the tactile rendering of textile surfaces. The approach proposed by HAPTEX consists of three parts: a model of the fabric describing its small scale physical and geometrical properties, a module capable of generating signals for the hardware and a module connecting the fabric's model with the signal generator. The latter module takes as input the finger's position and transforms the information contained in the fabric's model into appropriate signals.

Whole Haptic Interface

The separate force-feedback and the tactile components of the whole HAPTEX interface already represent significant advances with respect to the state of the art in terms of feedback accuracy and spatial stimulus distribution over the skin. But one of the main achievements of HAPTEX was the successful and smooth integration of the two force – and tactile rendering modalities and their associated hardware components. Distributed tactile stimulation (using a tactile rendering strategy which is designed to reproduce the sensation of a real surface) was combined with force-feedback for the first time. This integration was achieved in the first final demonstrator (see Fig. 3.42, bottom left), which is a unique system for the presentation of virtual textiles capable of delivering appropriate stimuli to the user.

Moreover, the second final demonstrator (see Fig. 3.42, bottom right) proved to have a very strong innovation potential. This demonstrator consisted of an actuated and sensorised wrist-grounded hand exoskeleton, connected to a sensorised mechanical tracker returning the absolute position/orientation of the proximal link of the hand exoskeleton with respect to the fixed frame of reference. The hand exoskeleton consisted of two actuated and sensorised finger exoskeletons (one for the index and one for the thumb) connected to a dorsal plate (proximal link of the hand exoskeleton) and secured to the palm of the hand through a glove like structure equipped with suitable belts and fastenings. All its components were designed to match the requirements of a modular haptic glove capable of rendering the haptic properties of light deformable objects at multiple contact points.

Milestones

The HAPTEX project has set important milestones in the research of multimodal interfaces for perceiving thin deformable objects and has achieved several breakthroughs.

Firstly, it produced an innovative working system which successfully synchronized a realistic visual representation of a deformable textile with appropriate kinesthetic and tactile stimuli on the thumb and index finger simultaneously (Fontana et al. 2007).

Secondly, the textile physical behavior, the tactile rendering and the force-feedback were computed by accurate mechanical models relying on physical parameters measured from real fabrics and synchronized in real time (Volino et al. 2007).

Thirdly, it generated a vast amount of expertise and know-how with a high educational impact, providing methodologies applicable for multimodal simulation of deformable objects (Magnenat-Thalmann et al. 2007b), thus paving the ground for further research on haptic simulation and interaction.

References

AATCC Technical Manual 2002, www.aatcc.org

Abbott N. J.: The Measurement of Stiffness in Textile Fabrics. Textile Research Journal, Vol. 21, 435–444 (1951)

Allerkamp D., Böttcher G., Wolter F. E., Brady A. C., Qu J., Summers I. R.: A vibrotactile approach to tactile rendering. The Visual Computer, Vol. 23, Issue 2, 97–108 (2007)

Askeland D. R., Phulé P. P.: The Science & Engineering of Materials. 5th edition, Thomson-Engineering, ISBN 0534553966 (2005)

Baraff D., Witkin A., Kass M.: Untangling Cloth. ACM Transactions on Graphics (ACM SIGGRAPH 2003), Vol. 22, 862–870 (2003)

Baraff D., Witkin A.: Large Steps in Cloth Simulation. Computer Graphics (SIGGRAPH'98 proceedings), ACM Press, 43–54 (1998)

Barbic J., James D. L.: Real-Time Subspace Integration for St.Venant-Kirchhoff Deformable Models. ACM Transactions on Graphics (ACM SIGGRAPH 2005 proceedings) (2005)

Bathe K. J.: Finite Element procedures. Prentice-Hall, Englewood Cliffs, NJ (1995)

Behre B.: Mechanical Properties of Textile Fabrics Part I: Shearing. Textile Research Journal, Vol. 31, Issue 2, 87–93 (1961)

Bianchi G., Solenthaler B., Székely G., Harders M.: Simultaneous Topology and Stiffness Identification for Mass-Spring Models Based on FEM Reference Deformations. Medical Image Computing and Computer-Assisted Intervention Proceedings, C. Barillot, Vol. 2, 293–301 (2004)

Bonet J., Wood R.: Nonlinear Continuum Mechanics for Finite Element Analysis. Cambridge University Press, Cambridge (1997)

Böttcher G., Allerkamp D., Wolter F. E.: Virtual Reality Systems Modelling Haptic Two-Finger Contact with Deformable Physical Surfaces. Proceedings of the International Conference on Cyberworlds 2007, 292–299 (2007)

Bottino A., Laurentini A., Scalabrin S.: Quantitatively Comparing Virtual and Real Draping of Clothes. International Conferences in Central Europe on Computer Graphics, Visualization and Computer Vision, WSCG, 63–70 (2001)

Breen D. E., House D. H., Wozny M. J.: Predicting the Drape of Woven Cloth using Interacting Particles, Computer Graphics (SIGGRAPH'94 proceedings), Glassner, 365–372 (1994)

Bridson R., Fedkiw R., Anderson J.: Robust Treatment of Collisions, Contact, and Friction for Cloth Animation. ACM Transactions on Graphics (ACM. SIGGRAPH 2002), 594–603 (2002)

Bro-Nielsen M., Cotin S.: Real-Time Volumetric Deformable Models for Surgery Simulation Using Finite Elements and Condensation, Eurographics 1996 Proceedings, ACM Press, 21–30 (1996)

Carignan M., Yang Y., Magnenat-Thalmann N., Thalmann D.: Dressing Animated Synthetic Actors with Complex Deformable Clothes, Computer Graphics (SIGGRAPH'92 proceedings), Addison-Wesley, Vol. 26, Issue 2, 99–104 (1992)

Choi K. J., Ko H. S.: Stable But Responsive Cloth, Computer Graphics (SIGGRAPH'02 Proceedings), Addison Wesley, 604–611 (2002)

Cohen J. D., Lin M. C., Manocha D., Ponamgi M. K.: I-COLLIDE: An Interactive and Exact Collision Detection System for Large-Scale Environments. Symposium of Interactive 3D Graphics Proceedings, 189–196 (1995)

Collier J. R., Collier B. J., O'Toole G., Sargand S. M.: Drape Prediction by Means of Finite Element Analysis. Journal of the Textile Institute, Vol. 82, Issue 1, 96–107 (1991)

Cooper D. N. E.: The Stiffness of Woven Textile. Journal of the Textile Institute, Vol. 51, T317–T335 (1960)

Cordier F., Magnenat-Thalmann N.: A Data-Driven Approach for Real-Time Clothes Simula-tion, Computer Graphics Forum, Vol. 24, Issue 2, 173–183 (2005)

Cordier F., Magnenat-Thalmann N.: Real-Time Animation of Dressed Virtual Humans. Computer Graphics Forum, Blackwell Publishing, Vol. 21, Issue 3, 327–336 (2002)

Cotin S., Delingette H., Ayache N.: Real-Time Elastic Deformations of Soft Tissues for Surgery Simulation. IEEE Transactions on Visualization and Computer Graphics, Vol. 5, Issue 1, 62–73 (1999)

Cusick G. E.: The Dependence of Fabric Drape on Bending and Shear Stiffness. Journal of the Textile Institute, Vol. 56, T596–T606 (1965)

Cusick G. E.: The Measurement of Fabric Drape. Journal of the Textile Institute, Vol. 59, 253–260 (1968)

Cusick G. E.: The Resistance of Fabrics to Shearing Forces. Journal of the Textile Institute, Vol. 52, 395–406 (1961)

Dahlberg B.: Mechanical Properties of Textile Fabrics, Part II: Buckling. Textile Research Journal, Vol. 31, Issue 2, 94–99 (1961)

De Boos A., Tester D.: FAST – Fabric Assurance by Simple Testing. Textile and Fiber Technology, Report No. WT92.02, ISBN 0 643 06025 1 (1994)

Debunne G., Desbrun M., Cani M. P., Barr A. H.: Dynamic Real-Time Deformations Using Space & Time Adaptive Sampling. Computer Graphics (SIGGRAPH'01 proceedings), Addison Wesley, 31–36 (2001)

Desbrun M., Schröder P., Barr A. H.: Interactive Animation of Structured Deformable Objects, Proceedings of Graphics Interface, A K Peters, 1–8 (1999)
Die Hohensteiner Institute. http://www.hohenstein.de. Accessed 30 November 2009
Dupont, Lycra. http://heritage.dupont.com. Accessed 30 November 2009
Eberhardt B., Etzmuss O., Hauth M.: Implicit-Explicit Schemes for Fast Animation with Particles Systems. Proceedings of the Eurographics Workshop on Computer Animation and Simulation, Springer-Verlag, 137–151 (2000)
Eberhardt B., Weber A., Strasser W.: A Fast Flexible Particle System Model for Cloth Draping. Computer Graphics and Applications, IEEE, Vol. 16, Issue 5, 52–59 (Sep 1996)
Eberhardt B., Weber A.: A Particle System Approach to Knitted Textiles. Computers & Graphics, Vol. 23, Issue 4, 599–560 (1999)
Eberhardt B., Weber A.: Modeling the Draping Behavior of Woven Cloth. MapleTech, Vol. 4, Issue 2, 25–31 (1997)
Eischen J. W., Deng S., Clapp T. G.: Finite Element Modeling and Control of Flexible Fabric Parts. Computer Graphics in Textiles and Apparel (IEEE Computer Graphics and Applications), IEEE Press, 71–80 (1996)
Etzmuss O., Gross J., Strasser W.: Deriving a Particle System from Continuum Mechanics for the Animation of Deformable Objects. IEEE Transactions on Visualization and Computer Graphics, IEEE Press, 538–550 (2003a)
Etzmuss O., Keckeisen M., Strasser W.: A Fast Finite Element Solution for Cloth Modeling. Proceedings of the 11th Pacific Conference on Computer Graphics and Applications, 244–251 (2003b)
Fontana M., Marcheschi S., Tarri F., Salsedo F., Bergamasco M., Allerkamp D., Böttcher G., Wolter F. E., Brady A. C., Qu J., Summers I. R.: Integrating Force and Tactile Rendering Into a Single VR System. Proceedings of the International Conference on Cyberworlds 2007, 277–284 (2007)
Fuhrmann A., Sobottka G., Gros C.: Distance Fields for Rapid Collision Detection in Physically-Based Modeling. Proceedings of GraphiCon, 58–65 (2003)
Fujimura K., Toriya H., Yamagushi K., Kunii T. L.: Octree Algorithms for Solid Modeling, Computer Graphics. Theory and Applications (InterGraphics'83 proceedings), Springer-Verlag, 96–110 (1983)
Gersak J., Sajn D., Bukosek V.: A Study of the Relaxation Phenomena in the Fabrics Containing Elastane Yarns. International Journal of Clothing Science and Technology, Vol. 17, Issue 3/4, 188–199 (2005)
Gilbert E. G., Foo C. P.: Computing the Distance Between General Convex Objects in 3D Space. IEEE Transactions on Robotics and Automation, Vol. 6, Issue 1, 53–61 (1990)
Gottschalk S., Lin M. C., Manocha D.: OBB-Tree: A Hierarchical Structure for Rapid Interference Detection. Computer Graphics (SIGGRAPH'96 proceedings), Addison-Wesley, 171–180 (1996)
Gould P.: Introduction to Linear Elasticity. 2nd edition, Springer (1993)
Govindaraj M., Garg A., Raheja A., Huang G., Metaxas D.: Haptic Simulation of Fabric Hand. Proceedings of Eurohap-tics Conference 2003, Vol. 1, 253–260 (2003)
Govindaraju N. K., Knott D., Jain N., Kabul I., Tamstorf R., Gayle R., Lin M., Manocha D.: Interactive Collision Detection between Deformable Models using Chromatic Decomposition. ACM Transactions on Graphics (ACM SIGGRAPH 2005), Vol. 24, Issue 3, 991–999 (2005)
Govindaraju N., Lin M., Manocha D.: Fast and Reliable Collision Detection Using Graphics Hardware. Proceedings of ACM VRST (2004)
Grinspun E., Hirani A. H., Desbrun M., Schröder P.: Discrete Shells. Eurographics Symposium on Computer Animation, 62–68 (2003)
Grosberg P., Swani N. M.: The Mechanical Properties of Woven Fabrics. Textile Research Journal, Vol. 36, 338–345 (1966)
Grzezczuk R., Terzopoulos D., Hinton G.: Neuroanimator: Fast Neural Network Emulation and Control of Physics-Based Models. Computer Graphics (SIGGRAPH'98 proceedings), Addison-Wesley, 9–20 (1998)

HAPTEX Consortium: Deliverable 4.3: Whole Haptic Interface Hardware. http://haptex.miralab.unige.ch/public/deliverables/HAPTEX-D4.3.pdf. Accessed 21 August 2008
HAPTEX Consortium: Deliverable 5.2: Final Demonstrator. http://haptex.miralab.unige.ch/public/deliverables/HAPTEX-D5.2.pdf. Accessed 21 August 2008
Hauth M., Etzmuss O.: A High Performance Solver for the Animation of Deformable Objects using Advanced Numerical Methods. Eurographics 2001 Proceedings, 137–151 (2001)
Hauth M., Strasser W.: Corotational Simulation of Deformable Solids, WSCG 2004 Proceedings, 137–145 (2004)
Heidelberger B., Teschner M., Gross M.: Detection of Collisions and Self-Collisions Using Image-Space Techniques. Journal of WSCG, Vol. 12, Issue 3, 145–152 (2004)
Heidelberger B., Teschner M., Gross M.: Realtime Volumetric Intersections of Deforming Objects. Proceedings of Vision, Modeling and Visualization, 461–468 (2003)
Held M., Klosowski J. T., Mitchell J. S. B.: Evaluation of Collision Detection Methods for Virtual Reality Fly-Throughs. Proceedings of the 7th Canadian Conference on Computational Geometry (1995)
Hubbard P. M.: Approximating Polyhedra with Spheres for Time-Critical Collision Detection. ACM Transactions on Graphics, Vol. 15, Issue 3, 179–210 (1996)
Hui C. L.: Neural Network Prediction of Human Psychological Perceptions of Fabric Hand. Textile Research Journal, Vol. 74 (2004)
Hutter M., Fuhrmann A.: Optimized Continuous Collision Detection for Deformable Triangle Meshes. Proceedings of WSCG '07, 25–32 (2007)
Instron. http://www.instron.us. Accessed 28 April 2008
Irving G., Teran J., Fedkiw R.: Invertible Finite Elements for Robust Simulation of Large Deformation. Eurographics Symposium on Computer Animation, 131–140 (2004)
Isshi T.: Bending Tester for Fibers, Yarns and Fabrics. Journal of the Textile Machinery Society of Japan, Vol. 3, Issue 2, 48–52 (1957)
James D., Pai D.: ArtDefo – Accurate Real-Time Deformable Objects. Computer Graphics (SIGGRAPH'99 proceedings), ACM Press, 65–72 (1999)
Johnson K. O., Yoshioka T. and Vega-Bermudez F.: Tactile Functions of Mechanoreceptive Afferents Innervating the Hand. Journal of Clinical Neurophysiology, Vol. 17, 539–558 (2000)
Johnson K. O.: The Roles and Functions of Cutaneous Mechanoreceptors. Current Opinion in Neurobiology, Vol. 11, 455–461 (2001)
Kang Y. M., Choi J. H., Cho H. G., Lee D. H., Park C. J.: Real-Time Animation Technique for Flexible and Thin Objects. WSCG'2000 Proceedings, 322–329 (2000)
Kawabata S.: The Standardization and Analysis of Hand Evaluation, 2nd edition. The Hand Evaluation and Standardization Committee, The Textile Machinery Society of Japan, Osaka (1980)
Kenkare N., May-Plumlee T.: Evaluation of Drape Characteristics in Fabrics. International Journal of Clothing Science and Technology, Vol. 17, Issue 2, 109–123 (2005)
Klosowski J. T., Held M., Mitchell J. S. B.: Efficient Collision Detection Using Bounding Volume Hierarchies of K-Dops. IEEE transactions on Visualization and Computer Graphics, Vol. 4, Issue 1 (1997)
Lafleur B., Magnenat-Thalmann N., Thalmann D.: Cloth Animation with Self-Collision Detection, IFIP conference on Modeling in Computer Graphics Proceedings, Springer-Verlag, 179–197 (1991)
Larsson T., Akenine-Möller T.: A Dynamic Bounding-Volume Hierarchy for Generalized Collision Detection. Computers and Graphics, Vol. 30, Issue 3, 451–460 (2006)
Leapfrog European Union. www.leapfrog-eu.org. Accessed 28 April 2008
Li Y.: The Science of Clothing Comfort. Journal of the Textile Institute, Textile Progress, Vol. 31, Issue 1/2 (1940)
Lindberg J., Dahlberg B.: Mechanical Properties of Textile Fabrics, Part III: Shearing and Buckling of Various Commercial Fabrics. Textile Research Journal, Vol. 31, Issue 2, 99–122 (1961)
Livesey R. G., Owen J. D.: Cloth Stiffness and Hysteresis in Bending. Journal of the Textile Institute, Vol. 55, Issue 10 (1964)

Loschek I.: Reclams Mode und Kostümlexikon. Philipp Reclam jun. GmbH & Co., Stuttgart, ISBN 3-15-010403-3 (1994)

Magnenat-Thalmann N., Volino P., Bonanni U., Summers I. R., Bergamasco M., Salsedo F., Wolter F. E.: From Physics-Based Simulation to the Touching of Textiles: The HAPTEX Project, The International Journal of Virtual Reality, Vol. 6, Issue 3, 35–44 (2007)

Magnenat-Thalmann N., Volino P., Bonanni U., Summers I. R., Brady A. C., Qu J., Allerkamp D., Fontana M., Tarri F., Salsedo F., Bergamasco M.: Haptic Simulation, Perception and Manipulation of Deformable Objects. In: Myszkowski K, Havran V (eds.) Eurographics 2007 – Tutorials. Prague, Eurographics Association, 1–22 (2007)

Mäkinnen M., Meinander H., Luible C., Magnenat-Thalmann N.: Influence of Physical Parameters on Fabric Hand. Proceedings of Workshop on Haptic and Tactile Perception of Deformable Objects, Hanover (2005)

Meyer M., Debunne G., Desbrun M., Barr A. H.: Interactive Animation of Cloth-like Objects in Virtual Reality. Journal of Visualization and Computer Animation, Wiley, Vol. 12, Issue 1, 1–12 (2001)

Mezger J., Kimmerle S., Etzmuss O.: Hierarchical Techniques in Collision Detection for Cloth Animation. Journal of WSCG, Vol. 11, Issue 2, 322–329 (2003)

Minazio P. G.: FAST – Fabric Assurance by Simple Testing. International Journal of Clothing Science and Technology, Vol. 7, Issue 2/3 (1995)

Mirtich B.: V-CLIP: Fast and Robust Polyhedral Collision Detection. ACM Transactions on Graphics (1998)

Muller M., Dorsey J., McMillan L., Jagnow R., Cutler B.: Stable Real-Time Deformations. Proceedings of the Eurographics Symposium on Computer Animation, 49–54 (2002)

Muller M., Gross M.: Interactive Virtual Materials, Proceedings of Graphics Interface. Canadian Human-Computer Communications Society, 239–246 (2004)

Nealen A., Müller M., Keiser R., Boxerman E., Carlson M.: Physically Based Deformable Models in Computer Graphics. Eurographics 05 State-of-the-Art Reports (2005)

Nesme M., Payan Y., Faure F.: Efficient, Physically Plausible Finite Elements. Eurographics 2005 Proceedings (short papers), 77–80 (2005)

O'Brien J., Hodgins J.: Graphical Modeling and Animation of Brittle Fracture. Computer Graphics (SIGGRAPH'99 proceedings), ACM Press, 137–146 (1999)

Otaduy M., Chassot O., Steinemann D., Gross M.: Balanced Hierarchies for Collision Detection Between Fracturing Objects. IEEE Virtual Reality (2007)

Palmer I. J., Grimsdale R. L.: Collision Detection for Animation using Sphere-Trees. Computer Graphics Forum, Vol. 14, 105–116 (1995)

Peirce F. T.: The Geometry of Cloth Structure. Journal of the Textile Institute, Vol. 28, T45–T96 (1937)

Peirce F. T.: The Handle of Cloth as a Measurable Quantity. Journal of the Textile Institute, Vol. 21, 377–416 (1930)

Picinbono G., Delingette H., Ayache N.: Non-Linear Anisotropic Elasticity for Real-Time Surgery Simulation. Graphical Models, Vol. 65, Issue 5, 305–321 (2003)

Press W.H., Flannery B.P., Tukolsky S.A., Vetterling W.T.: Numerical Recipes in C: The Art of Scientific Computing. 2nd edition, Cambridge University Press (1992)

Proske U.: What is the Role of Muscle Receptors in Proprioception? Muscle Nerve, Wiley Periodicals, Vol. 31, Issue 6, 780–787 (2006)

Redon S., Kheddar A., Coquillart S.: Fast Continuous Collision Detection Between Rigid Bodies. Computer Graphics Forum (Proceedings of Eurographics'02) (2002)

Rowe M. J., Tracey D. J., Mahns D.A., Sahai V., Ivanusic J. J.: Mechanosensory Perception: are There Contributions From Bone-Associated Receptors?, Clinical and Experimental Pharmacology and Physiology, Blackwell Publishing, Vol. 32, Issue 1–2, 100–108 (2006)

Stylios G.: New Measurement Technologies for Textiles and Clothing. International Journal of Clothing Science and Technology, Vol. 17, Issue 3/4, 135–149 (2005)

Sud A., Govindaraju N., Gayle R., Kabul I., Manocha D.: Fast Proximity Computation Among Deformable Models Using Discrete Voronoi Diagrams. ACM Transactions on Graphics (SIGGRAPH 2006 proceedings), Vol. 25, Issue 3, 1144–1153 (2006)

Summers I. R., Brady A. C., Syed M., Chanter C. M.: Design of Array Stimulators for Synthetic Tactile Sensations. Proceedings of the World Haptics'05, 586–587 (2005)

Terzopoulos D., Platt J., Barr A., Fleischer K.: Elastically Deformable Models, SIGGRAPH '87: Proceedings of the 14th annual Conference on Computer Graphics and Interactive Techniques, ACM, 205–214 (1987)

Teschner M., Kimmerle S., Heidelberger B., Zachmann G., Raghupathi L., Fuhrmann A., Cani M. P., Faure F., Magnenat-Thalmann N., Strasser W., Volino P.: Collision Detection for Deformable Objects, Computer Graphics Forum, Vol. 24, Issue 1, 61–81 (2005)

Timoshenko S. P., Goodier J. N.: Theory of elasticity. 3rd edition, McGraw-Hill (1970)

Van Den Bergen G.: Efficient Collision Detection of Complex Deformable Models Using AABB Trees. Journal of Graphics Tools, Vol. 2, Issue 4, 1–14 (1997)

Volino P., Courchesne M., Magnenat-Thalmann N.: Versatile and Efficient Techniques for Simulating Cloth and Other Deformable Objects Computer Graphics (SIGGRAPH'95 proceedings), Addison-Wesley, 137–144 (1995)

Volino P., Davy P., Bonanni U., Luible C., Magnenat-Thalmann N., Mäkinen M., Meinander M.: From Measured Physical Parameters to the Haptic Feeling of Fabric. The Visual Computer, Vol. 23, Issue 2, 133–142 (2007)

Volino P., Magnenat-Thalmann N.: Accurate Garment Prototyping and Simulation. Computer-Aided Design & Applications, CAD Solutions, Vol. 2, Issue 5, 645–654 (2005)

Volino P., Magnenat-Thalmann N.: Developing Simulation Techniques for an Interactive Clothing System, Virtual Systems and Multimedia (VSMM'97 proceedings), Geneva, Switzerland, 109–118 (1997)

Volino P., Magnenat-Thalmann N.: Efficient Self-Collision Detection on Smoothly Discretised Surface Animation Using Geometrical Shape Regularity. Computer Graphics Forum (Eurographics'94 proceedings), Blackwell Publishers, Vol. 13, Issue 3, 155–166 (1994)

Volino P., Magnenat-Thalmann N.: Implicit Midpoint Integration and Adaptive Damping for Efficient Cloth Simulation. Computer Animation and Virtual Worlds, Wiley, Vol. 16, Issues 3–4, 163–175 (2005)

Volino P., Magnenat-Thalmann N.: Simple Linear Bending Stiffness in Particle Systems. SIGGRAPH-Eurographics Symposium on Computer Animation 2006 Proceeding, 101–105 (2006)

Wang X., Devarajan V.: 1D and 2D Structured Mass-Spring Models with Preload. The Visual Computer, Springer, Vol. 21, Issue 7, 429–448 (2005)

Webb R. C., Gigante M. A.: Using Dynamic Bounding Volume Hierarchies to improve Efficiency of Rigid Body Simulations. Communicating with Virtual Worlds (CGI'92 proceedings), 825–841 (1992)

Werner H. M., Magnenat-Thalmann N., Thalmann D.: User Interface for Fashion Design, Graphics, Design and Visualization (ICCG'93 proceedings), 165–172 (1993)

Yamaguchi K., Kunii T. L., Fujimura K.: Octree Related Data Structures and Algorithms. IEEE Computer Graphics and Applications, 53–59 (1984)

Yang Y., Magnenat-Thalmann N.: An Improved Algorithm for Collision Detection in Cloth Animation with Human Body, Computer Graphics and Applications (Pacific Graphics'93 proceedings), Vol. 1, 237–251 (1993)

Zachmann G., Weller R.: Kinetic Bounding Volume Hierarchies for Deforming Objects. ACM International Conference on Virtual Reality Continuum and its Applications (2006)

Zhang X., Redon S., Lee M., Kim Y. J.: Continuous Collision Detection for Articulated Models Using Taylor Models and Temporal Culling, ACM Transactions on Graphics (SIGGRAPH 2007 Proceedings), Vol. 26, Issue 3 (2007)

Zhou N., Ghosh T. K.: On-Line Measurement of Fabric Bending Behavior: Background, Need and Potential Solutions. International Journal of Clothing Science and Technology, Vol. 10, Issue 2, 143–156 (1998)

Zhuang Y., Canny J.: Haptic Interaction with Global Deformations. Proceedings of the IEEE International Conference on Robotics and Automation, IEEE Press (2000)

Chapter 4
Designing and Animating Patterns and Clothes

Abstract Clothing simulation tools are used in the garment industry to design and prototype garments before the manufacturing process. Designers create 3D clothes based on 2D patterns which are either imported from CAD systems or created manually. This chapter describes the 3D tailoring process, from the initial creation of 2D patterns to the sewing around a virtual mannequin in 3D space. This process is then presented on a case study showing the making of the award winning film "High Fashion in Equations".

4.1 Introduction

Clothing simulation tools are frameworks, which fit the needs of the garment industry, concentrating on the simulation and visualization features. The frameworks integrate innovative tools, aimed for efficiency and quality in the process of garment design and prototyping, taking advantage of state-of-the-art algorithms from the field of mechanical simulation, animation and rendering. Simulation tools allow designers to create 3D clothes based on 2D patterns. Patterns can be either imported from CAD systems (Lectra, Gerber) or be manually created. For the tailoring process, applications emulate the real world garment-production processes: the patterns are initially designed and cut in 2D space, placed around a virtual mannequin in 3D space, sewn together to make a complete clothing. Finally the 3D garment is simulated according to physical and mechanical fabric properties in the virtual environment.

The overall visual appearance of a garment (real or virtual) is influenced by two main components: The shape of the 3D garment, determined by the corresponding 2D pattern and the fabric material used which behavior is influenced by its mechanical and physical properties (Fig. 4.1). In the following the single steps, necessary for the creation of a virtual garment are explained.

N. Magnenat-Thalmann (ed.), *Modeling and Simulating Bodies and Garments*,
DOI 10.1007/978-1-84996-263-6_4,

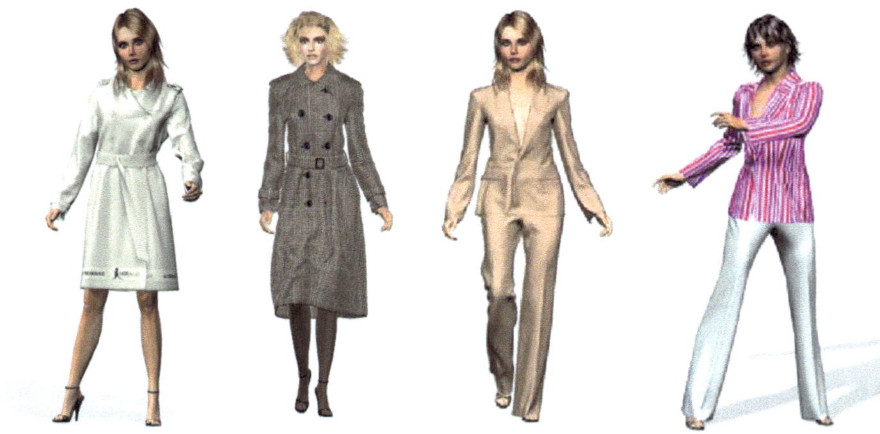

Fig. 4.1 Four examples of virtually animated garments (Miralab – University of Geneva)

4.2 Pattern Design

The 2D pattern creation is a precise handiwork. Having the desired 3D shape in mind, a flat pattern is drawn by skilled experts according to pattern construction rules. There are several ways to obtain the two-dimensional description of the 3D garment. The most traditional method is the construction using a ruler and a pencil on paper.

4.2.1 Digitalization

For a use in 3D applications, the traditionally constructed 2D paper pattern needs to be digitized on a digitalization board (Fig. 4.2). For the digitalization, the paper pattern is fixed on the board. Subsequently, the outlines and the construction lines of the 2D pattern are traced with a special mouse. Different mouse buttons allow the creation of different points and markers. Applying this method, the shapes of the single pattern pieces are copied to the CAD software and consequently, the 2D pattern can be edited such as an electronical pattern and exported to the 3D application (Fig. 4.3).

4.2.2 Import from CAD Software

Most apparel companies develop their 2D pattern directly with CAD software's, allowing an easy editing of the shapes. Moreover, the pattern pieces are part of the entire garment collection planning system. Thus, the garments designs are handled inside the CAD software on a high technological level. Garment styles can be easily copied and altered for the creation of new silhouettes (Fig. 4.4).

4.2.3 Extraction of the Outer Shell Pattern Pieces

In the simulation software, the seam allowances are generally not simulated. Therefore, only the 2D pattern outer shell is needed. The seam allowances can be either removed inside the CAD software or inside the 3D simulation application (Fig. 4.5).

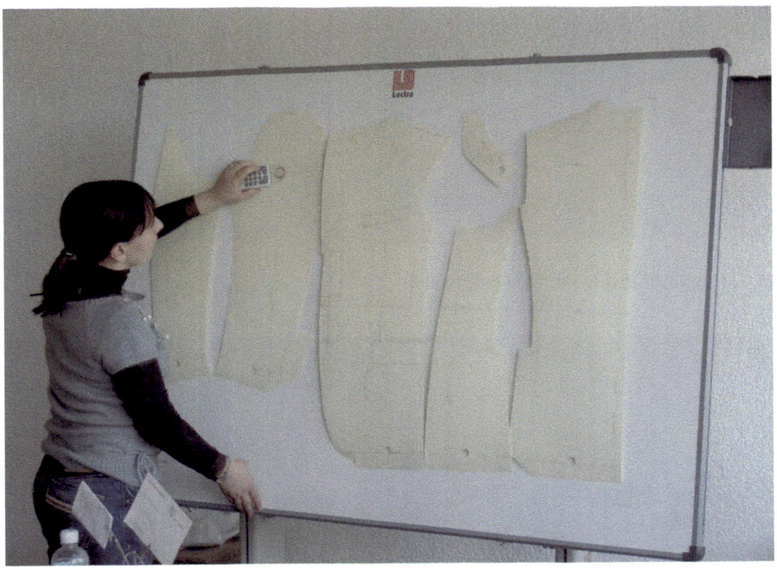

Fig. 4.2 2D pattern digitalization process

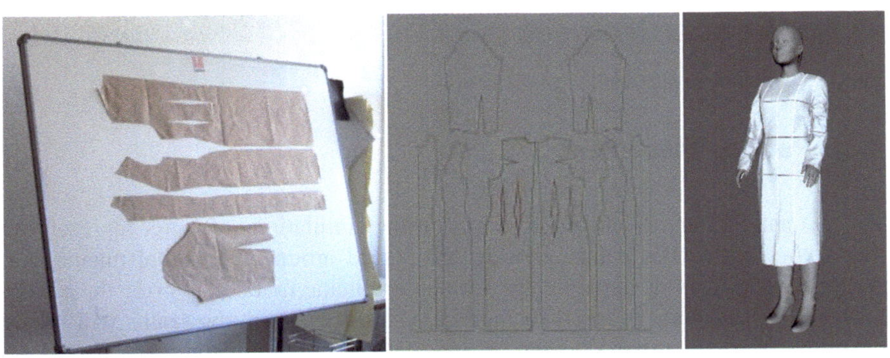

Fig. 4.3 Digitalization process: from the paper pattern (*left*) to the digitized pattern (*center*) and the virtual dress (*right*)

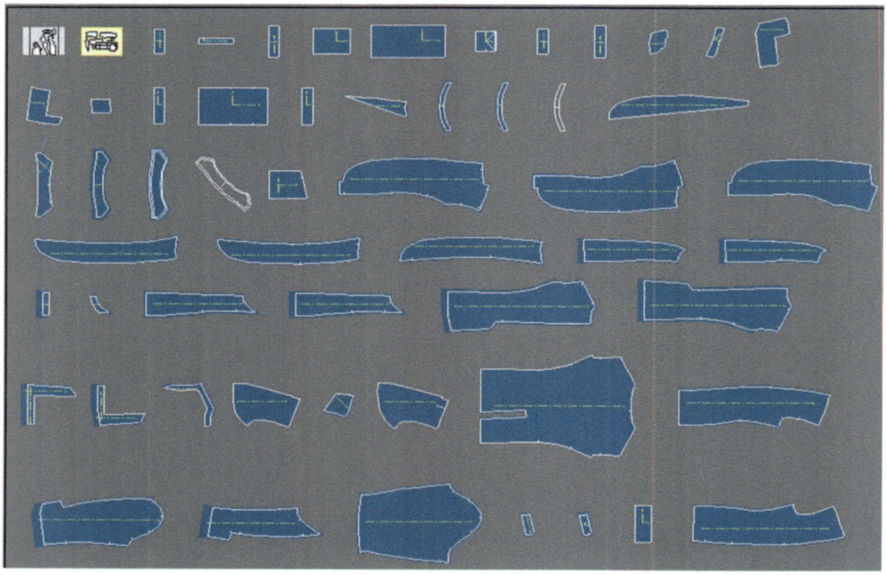

Fig. 4.4 2D pattern inside the CAD software

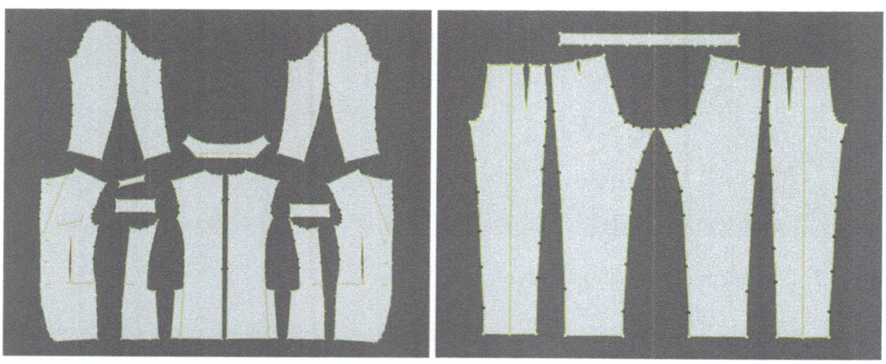

Fig. 4.5 Outer shell pattern of a men costume

4.3 Pattern Placement

The 2D patterns are displayed on a grid in the simulation software, representing the cloth surface. The planar patterns are placed around the virtual mannequin. A manual placement is implemented with an automatic function to bring the pattern to the closest position to the body surface. Considering that the seams will gather the edges of each pattern together, an approximate initial positioning is necessary. The space between two seam lines should be as small as possible in order to accelerate the process and to obtain a precise final garment (Fig. 4.6). Through the

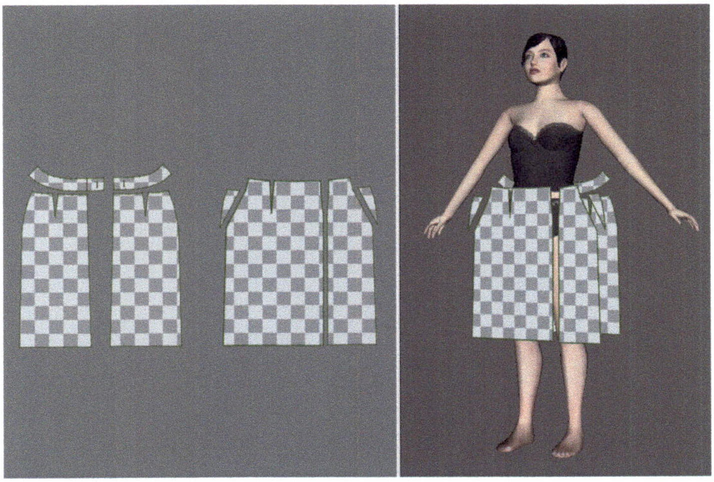

Fig. 4.6 2D pattern placement

collision detection, small initial problems can be automatically solved. It is preferable that the patterns do not interpenetrate itself and the body initially.

Further, a fully automatic placement method is available in the simulation software. It works according to a placement file, which has been created previously from a similar garment positioning. However the automatic placement is only recommended for serial garments with similar pattern pieces.

4.4 Seaming

After the placement of the patterns around the virtual mannequin, the seaming can be executed. In the simulation application the seams are indicated with red lines (Fig. 4.7). The seams are forcing the patterns to approach and to pull the matching pattern together during the simulation.

Several types of seams, which are available, describe various ways of how two surfaces are connected (closed mesh or open). Several seam parameters are available in order to imitate different seam characteristics.

4.5 Fabric Properties

The applied virtual fabric is composed in two components. On the one hand, the visual information of a textile is needed in the form of a texture map. This texture map should be a good quality picture of the fabric, showing the smallest repeat. On the other hand, the mechanical and physical parameters have to be applied to the

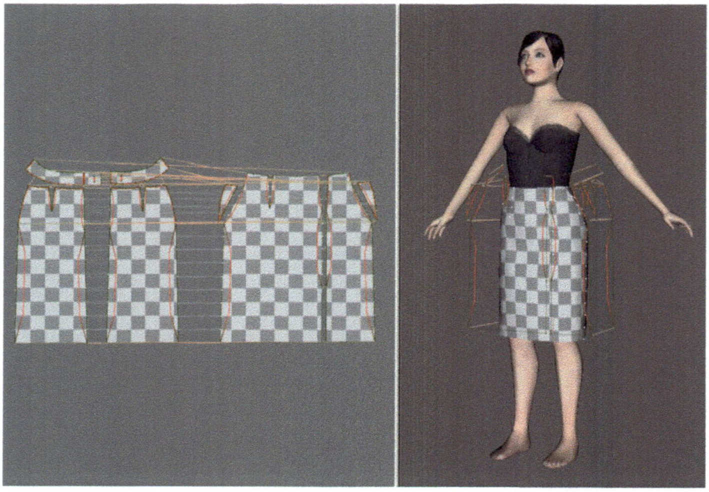

Fig. 4.7 Skirt with seams

garment at this stage. Since only precisely computed fabric characteristics can visualize different fabric qualities, their correct derivation from real fabric characteristics plays an important role (also see Chapter 3 about the measurement and parameter derivation).

4.6 Garment Fitting

Once the texturing and garment properties setting is completed the "fitting" of a garment can be executed by calling a mechanical simulation, which is forcing the surfaces to approach along the seam lines. The surface is deforming according to the shape of the body. The simulation engine first uses a simplified mechanical model, which is optimized in speed by leaving the physical parameters and environment parameters behind the calculation. After this first simulation, where the garment is fast approached to the shape of the body, a second mechanical model is taken for the actual simulation. This simulation is executed until the fabric is dynamically stabilized in a static position (Fig. 4.8).

The realistic clothing animation is simulated according to the movement of the virtual actor. This is possible thanks to the collision detection and friction with the surface of the body. The adjustments of simulation parameters can be different from those used during the process of seaming and assembling of the garment. Mechanical simulation gives the realism to the animation of clothing on the virtual mannequin.

In general, for the animation of clothing on virtual characters, the Vicon Motion Tracking System is used to record realistic body posture and fashion walks. All kind of movements can be simulated with state of the art simulation applications, from simple fashion walks to complex fitting movements (Figs. 4.9–4.12).

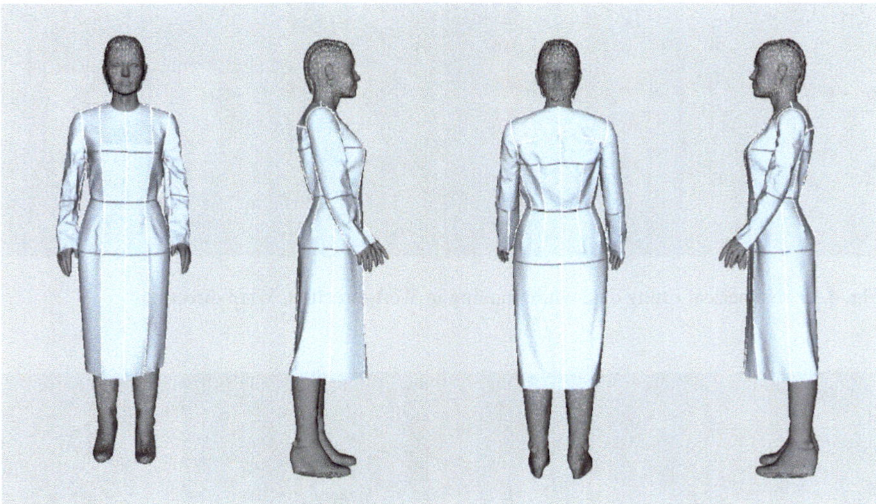

Fig. 4.8 Virtual static fitting

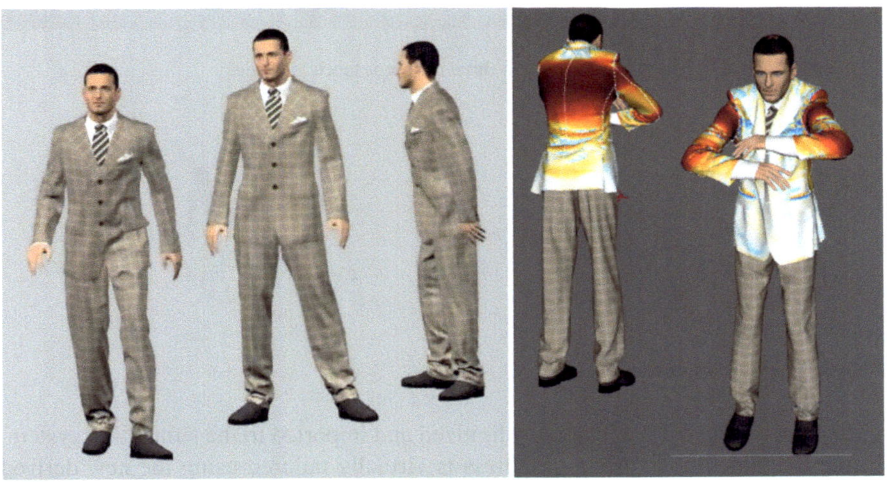

Fig. 4.9 Virtual prototyping of men suits visualizing numerical fitting data

4.7 Comparison of Real and Virtual Fitting Processes

Subsequently, an entire garment prototyping process is performed, comparing the real procedures with the virtual simulated ones. For the prototyping experiment the real mannequin is scanned with a body scanner to obtain an accurate virtual 3D body model. From the scan, exact body measurements are obtained, which are used for the construction of a real "made to measure" 2D pattern and dress. For the corresponding

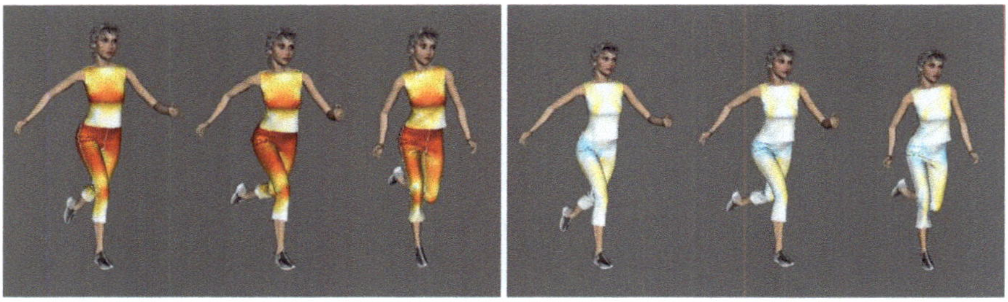

Fig. 4.10 Numerical fitting data while running in Weft-direction, Warp direction

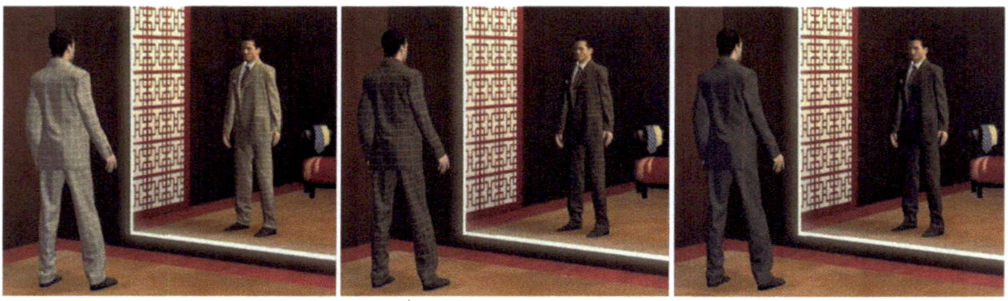

Fig. 4.11 Virtual try on of a men suits in three different fabric qualities

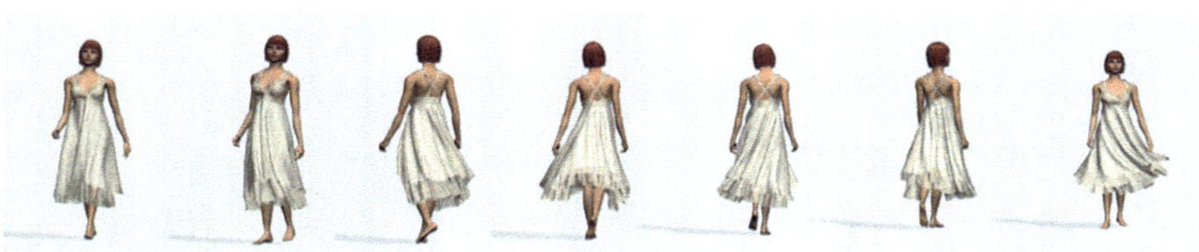

Fig. 4.12 Animated dress

virtual dress, the real 2D pattern is digitized and imported to the simulation system. Inside the simulation system, the dress is virtually tailored using the new derived fabric parameters. Afterwards, both the real and the virtual fitting procedures are performed in parallel and are compared.

A female mannequin is chosen for the prototyping experiment. The person is scanned with a body scanner, wearing underwear and shoes. As the underwear and shoes are influencing the body silhouette and posture, the same underwear and shoes are worn later on during the real fitting process. The body scanner automatically returns a predefined set of body measurements. Therefrom, the most important, necessary for the 2D pattern construction are retained. Out of this data, a simple, straight and close fitted dress is designed, customized for the mannequin's body. A standard 2D pattern construction method is applied. The real dress is tailored out of a simple cotton material. Before the assembly of the virtual dress, the 2D pattern is digitized (see Section 4.2.1).

In the following, the real garment behavior is directly compared with the virtual simulation. For each dress one or several movements are applied. The comparison stated a good visual correlation for the real and the virtual garments for the six tested fabrics (Figs. 4.13–4.18).

4.7.1 Physical Precision of the Simulation Result

In dynamic garment simulations, important additional error margins influence the simulation result, which are related to the body animation. In order to virtually animate the digital mannequin, several procedures are applied, where each of them adds some kind of inaccuracy to the virtual clone. Among them, the three main factors are the following:

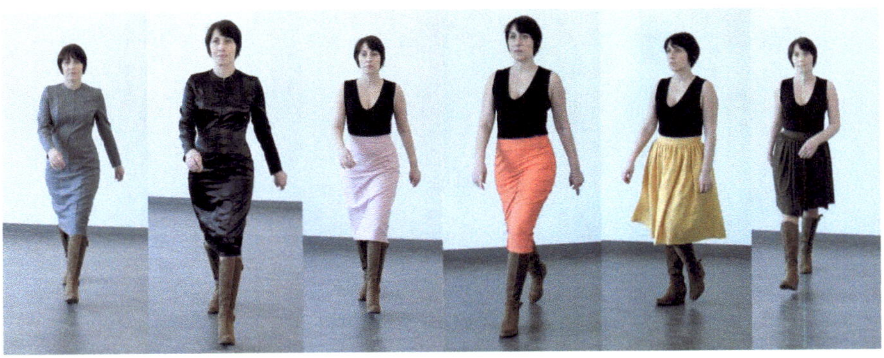

Fig. 4.13 Various garments and used fabrics: grey gabardine, black satin, pink flannel, orange weft-knit, yellow linen, brown weft-knit terry fabric

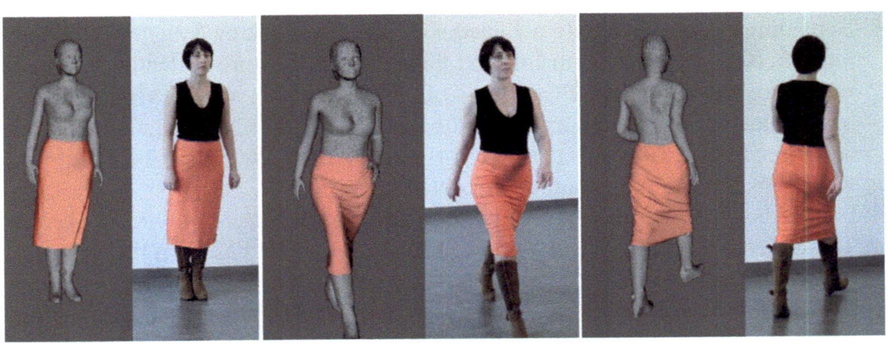

Fig. 4.14 Virtual and real orange weft-knit jersey skirt

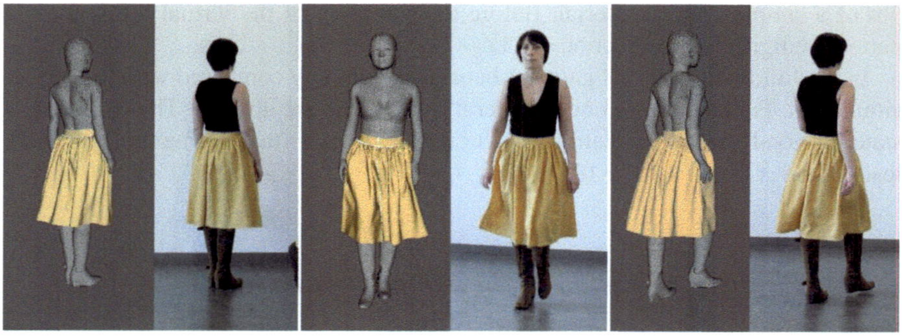

Fig. 4.15 Virtual and real yellow linen skirt

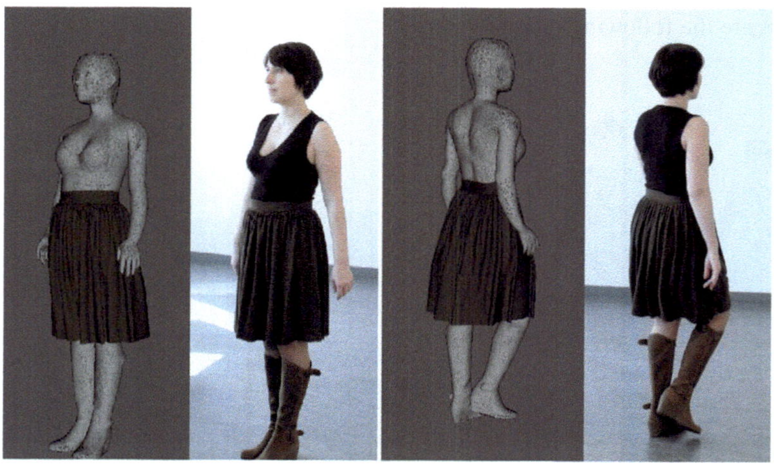

Fig. 4.16 Virtual and real brown weft-knit terry fabric skirt

- Body animations are mainly obtained with Motion Tracking Systems. The body movement is recorded with infrared cameras that capture reflecting markers, which are placed on significant parts of the body. However, due to instabilities of the markers during the recording, the obtained movement data is not 100% accurate. Inaccuracies of up to 4 cm (Leardini et al. 2005) can be comprises, what corresponds to one entire garment size step.
- For the body animation, the 3D mesh needs to be attached to a virtual Skelton. The dimension of the virtual Skelton is, however, again based on the imprecise motion capturing data.
- In order to finally animate the 3D body, the mesh has to be attached to the virtual Skeleton. This so called skinning process is made by hand and therefore, comprises additional inaccuracies.

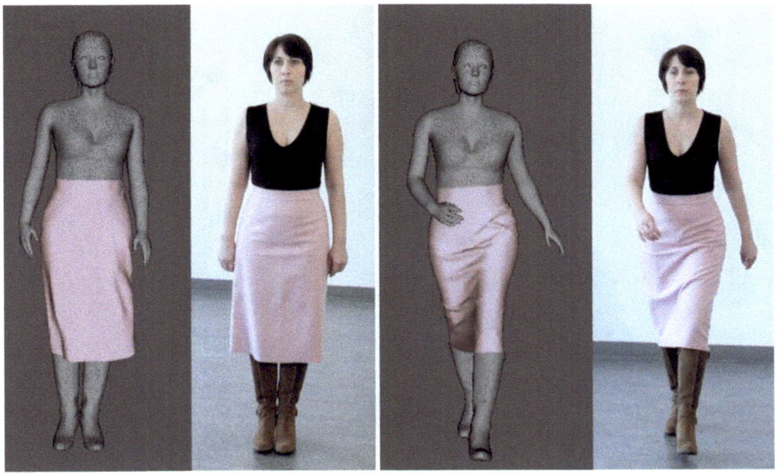

Fig. 4.17 Virtual and real pink flannel skirt

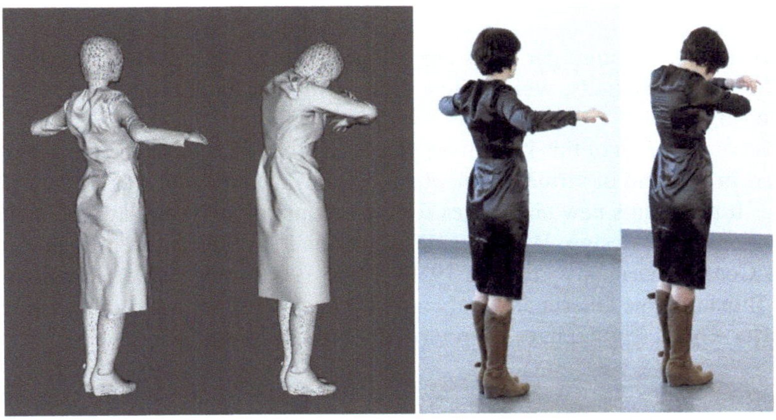

Fig. 4.18 Virtual and real black satin dress

4.8 The Making of the Award Winning Film: High Fashion in Equations

4.8.1 Introduction

Tailored out of exquisite materials and artful designed patterns, high fashion garments constitute the most sophisticated kind of clothes. The unique manufactured pieces, only affordable for a small circle of clientele, are not only envelopes for the human body, but artworks, visualizing cultural aspects, tendencies and trends.

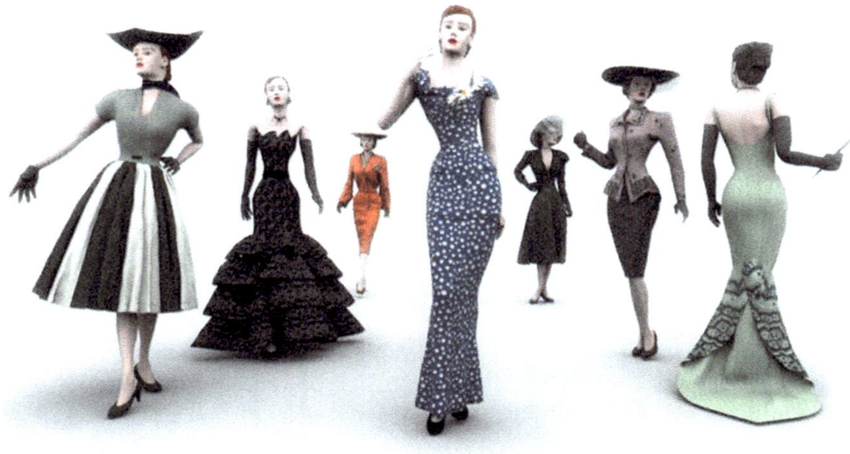

Fig. 4.19 Garment examples of high fashion in equation

Historical haute couture garments are characterized by an additional aspect: Time specific garment details, which allow their affiliation to certain époques, become visible (Fig. 4.19).

The computation of this kind of art pieces can thus be seen as the most challenging part in the field of virtual garment simulations, an area that was not touched on before. It represents new challenges for the computation system as well as for the realization of the design. With the 3D animation "High Fashion in Equations" 18 Haute Couture garments from the 1950s to the 1960s after fashion drawings from Marc Bohan, Serge Guérin and Hubert de Givenchy, former assistants of the Swiss couturier Robert Piguet, have been virtually brought to life.

4.8.2 Robert Piguet

Robert Piguet opened his Salon in 1933 in Paris, even so the Haute Couture ateliers generally suffered from the World Economic Crises at that time. Piguet himself was an excellent tailor. For the creative work Robert Piguet hired young talented designers such as Christian Dior, Marc Bohan, Serge Guerin and Hubert de Givenchy. In the 1930s, female and soft garment silhouettes were fashionable. During the World War Second, textile rationings obligated the creators to design more practical and simple garment pieces in Europe and the Haute Couture was almost completely disrupted. First post war clothes were still affected by austerity. Shapes were Victorian with broad shoulders and just knee-covered hems. In the 1940s feminine garment shapes re-conquered the fashion scene with the so called "New Look" including wide skirts and large material consumptions. The gowns of Piguet have

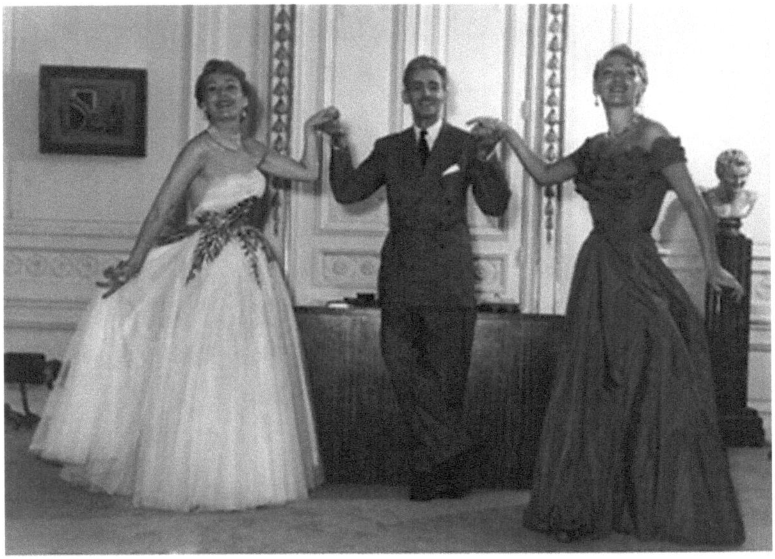

Fig. 4.20 Haute couture designer Robert Piguet with mannequins

been famous for a discrete elegance, appreciated by wealthy clients like aristocratic woman and artists (Fig. 4.20).

4.8.3 Inspiration

Fashion drawings are the original medium for the communication of new ideas about garment designs. The meaning of an aesthetic fashion drawing was always a different one as of for example a technical drawing: it is not only an information vehicle but can be seen as an artwork, visualizing also cultural aspects of a garment, corresponding to certain époques. Designers are characterized by their particular drawing styles, visible also in the different type of sketches of Dior, Castillo, Bohan, Givenchy and Guérin. Those sketches constitute excellent indication of the artistic goal searched by the designer. The sketches give some form of artistic life to the piece of clothing. The fashion drawing can be seen as an anticipatory vision in the designer's mind (Fig. 4.21).

However, shown in only two dimensions, a fashion drawing leaves a lot of space for individual interpretation of a garment in three dimensions. New computer graphics tools give the user the freedom to visualize the real world virtually in a realistic or a completely abstract way. This freedom allowed multiple virtual interpretations of the fashion drawings from Robert Piguet; the sketches could be either transformed into a very realistic virtual garment visualizing small details or into an abstract cloth related only to the idea of the designer. The final aesthetic of the

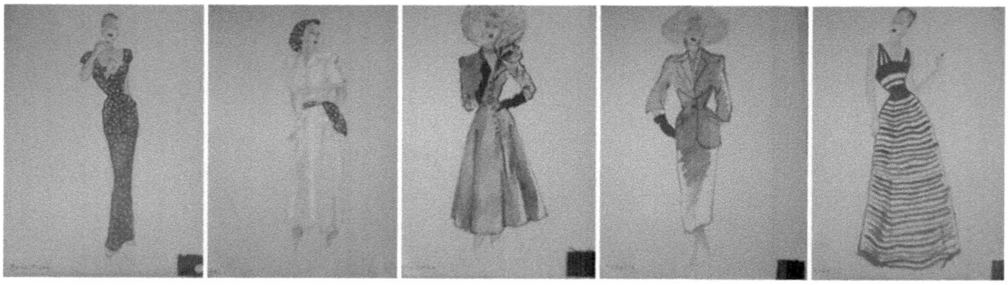

Fig. 4.21 Fashion drawings from Hubert de Givenchy

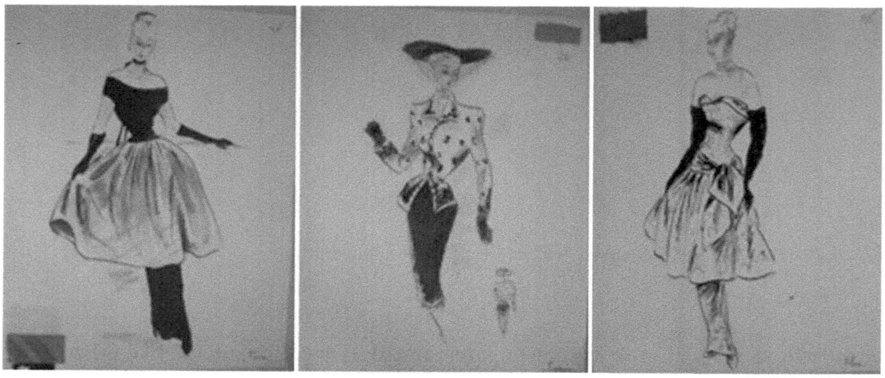

Fig. 4.22 Fashion drawings from Marc Bohan

virtual haute couture garments consisted in a balancing act between artificiality (towards the sketch) and realism (towards the real garments) (Fig. 4.22).

4.8.4 Design and Implementation

The overall visual appearance of a garment (real or virtual) is influenced by two main components: The shape of the 3D garment, determined by the corresponding 2D pattern and the fabric material used which behavior is influenced by its mechanical and physical properties (Fig. 4.23).

4.8.4.1 Unlimited Parameters for Virtual Representations

Shown in two-dimension from only one side, a sketch leaves a lot of space for individual interpretation of the garment in three-dimension (real or virtual). However, the interpretation in the form of a real tailored garment is limited by the morphology of the human body.

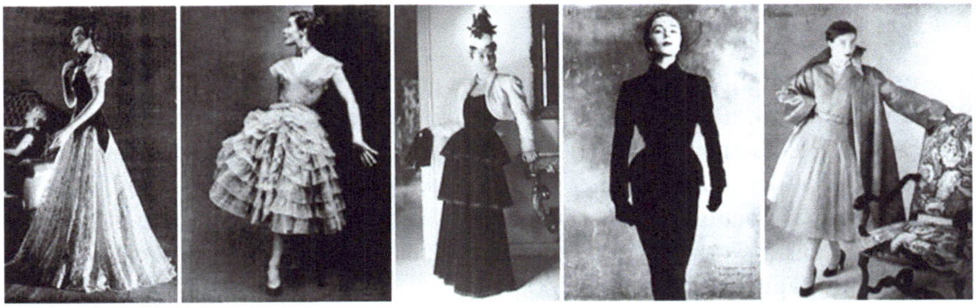

Fig. 4.23 Various designs from Robert Piguet

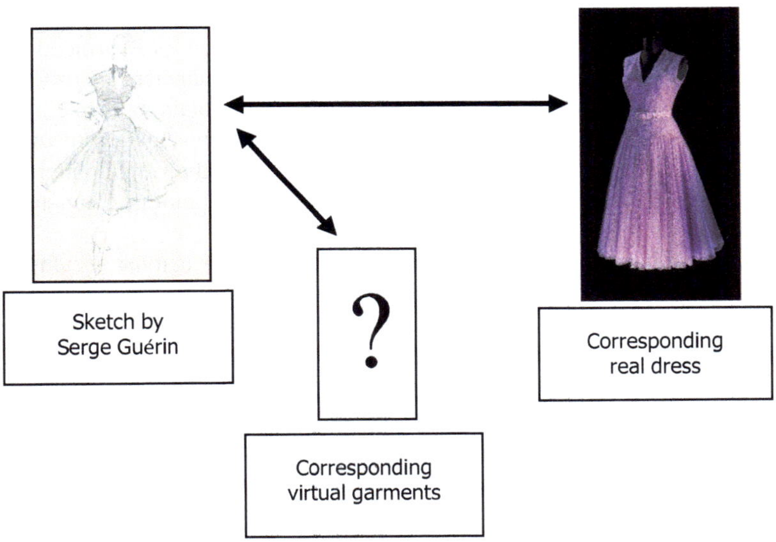

Fig. 4.24 The look of the virtual garment has to be found out of unlimited parameters

Virtual garments are composed of unlimited parameters. Thanks to developments in 3D Computer Graphics the real world can be completely imitated with graphics tools, giving the user the freedom to visualize the real world virtually in a realistic or a completely abstract way.

Regarding the project of Robert Piguet, this freedom allows thousands of different virtual interpretations of the Robert Piguet fashion drawings. The sketches could be either transformed into a very realistic virtual garment visualizing small details or into an abstract cloth related only to the idea of the Designer (Fig. 4.24).

4.8.4.2 Design of 2D Patterns

The creation of high fashion 2D patterns is a precise handwork. Having the desired 3D shape in mind, a flat pattern is drawn by skilled experts according to pattern construction rules. Therefore, ancient garments of that period have been studied for a better comprehension of former pattern making methods (Steele 2000). For the design of the 2D pattern, correct assembly, seaming and final animation of those complex virtual artworks, a highly versatile virtual garment design system was used (Volino and Magnenat-Thalmann 2005).

This virtual garment creation software imitates the real world tailoring process: the patterns are initially designed and cut in 2D space, placed around a virtual mannequin in 3D space, sewn together to make a completed clothing, and finally simulated according to the physical properties of the fabric and its environment. During the animation, the garment follows the movement of the virtual mannequin. Correct simulation parameters must be found out of multiple possibilities. This high standard simulation tools have been designed for the exact virtual prototyping of garments, but can also be used for visualization processes, where the input parameters are different.

To take a 2D pattern as a base is the simplest way to obtain a precise, exact and measurable description of a 2D surface, which is the representation of the virtual fabric. One garment is composed of several 2D surfaces, the single pattern pieces. Fashionizer is basically an editor of Polygons representing clothing in a number of 2D Polygons, connected by seam lines.

To derive the exact 2D pattern shape from the two-dimensional sketch, first the drawing needs to be interpreted by imaging it as a detailed 3D garment. Having the desired 3D shape in mind, the 2D pattern can be designed according to pattern construction rules. The dimensions of the 2D patterns are determined by the size of the body to be dressed. Would the original 2D patterns of the sketches have been available, they could have been digitized on a digitalization board and the obtained electronic data directly imported into Fashionizer from the CAD System and modified according to the size of the mannequin (Fig. 4.25).

Today's pattern construction methods are also affected by new developments in the textile and textile processing field. For instance elastic materials such as Lycra, which were only introduced on the textile market in 1962, suddenly allowed the production of tight fitted garments, without the need of complicated 2D pattern shapes. This progress of technology over the past 60 years needed to be considered in the creation of the 2D pattern for the Robert Piguet gowns, as it influences the global fit and appearance of a garment. The comfortability of a garment, what also comes from new elastic materials today, needed to be guaranteed completely by a comfortable cut of 2D pattern in that time.

4.8.4.3 Fabric Material

Since only precisely computed fabric characteristics can visualize the exquisite fabric qualities of high fashion garments, their correct derivation from real fabric characteristics plays an important role. Information on the fabrics used for those

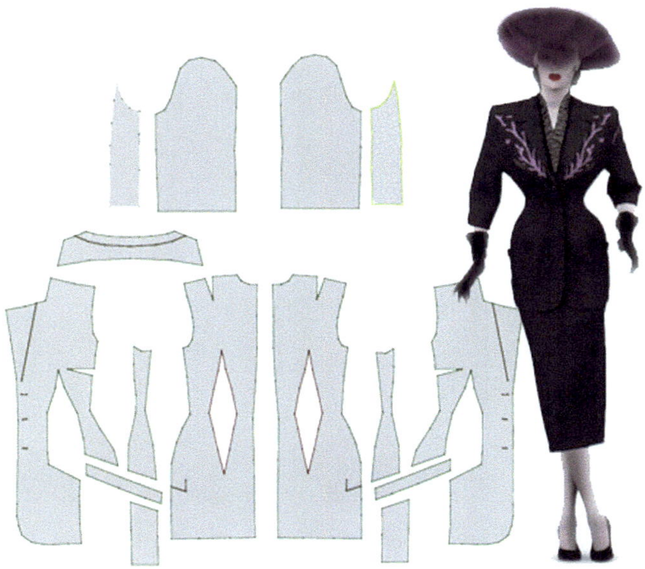

Fig. 4.25 Creation of 2d patterns for a jacket

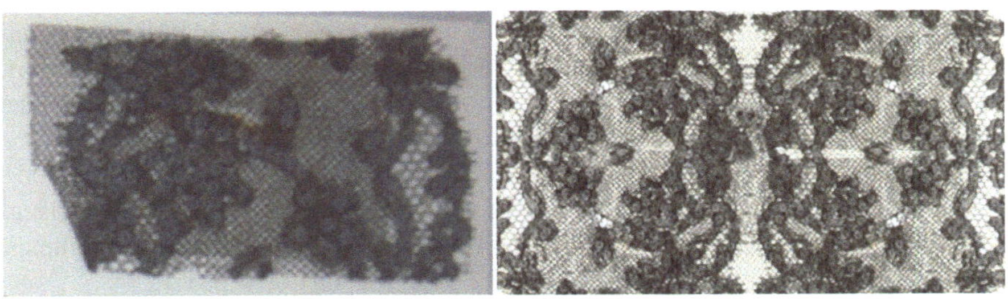

Fig. 4.26 Real texture on the sketch and optimized texture for mapping

designs was limited to material descriptions regarding structure and fiber compositions. Therefore, similar fabric materials have been chosen and measured with fabric characterization experiments, to obtain strain–stress curves for the main mechanical and physical fabric properties, which were fitted with polynomial splines (Fig. 4.26).

Textile color and quality information was additionally found in hand written form on the original sketches. Surprisingly this information did not correspond in some cases to the fabric, attached to the drawing. The small fabric swatches are almost 60 years old and the original shade had discolored over time. Priority was then given to the hand written information on the sketch and similar fabrics were searched from a fabric library. The chosen fabrics were photographed and prepared in a repetitive way for texture mapping. In addition typical buttons and buckles from the 1940s were photographed to be mapped as accessories (Fig. 4.27).

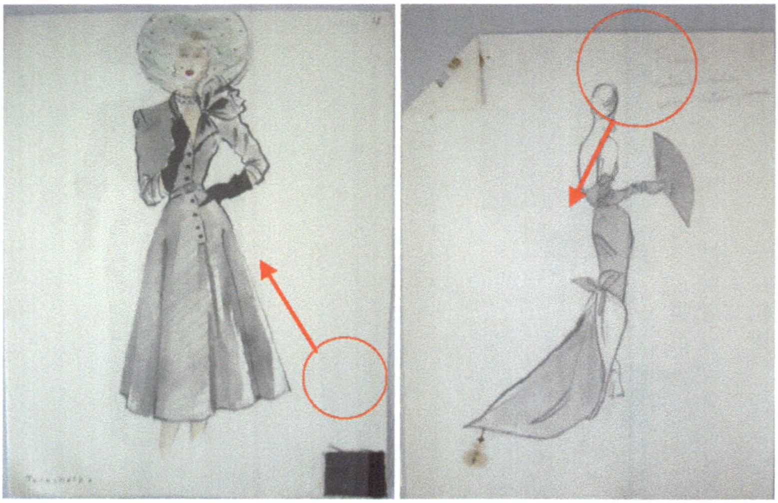

Fig. 4.27 Drawing and fabric information are different and hand written fabric information

4.8.4.4 Intended Aesthetic

For the production of the animation "High fashion in Equations", the overall visual appearance had to match the scenario. The accuracy aspect was less important. First, the dimension of the character was not limited to realistic body dimensions anymore and could be designed and modeled in an abstract way that fits to the common concept. The 2D patterns were then designed according to the abstracted body dimension of the mannequin. The fitting of the garments was affected by the visual appearance and not by the fit to a certain size. All possibilities and parameter, depending on the level of abstractness, can be imagined (Fig. 4.28).

The original drawings of the Piguet gowns from the 1940s are characterized by their specific aesthetics that transport the cultural information about the post war period. Garments, accessories and also hairstyles are conformed to trends of respective epochs. To make time tendencies in clothing visible, exact details of a cloth have to be shown, since they describe their affiliation to a certain time. To make these components visible a realistic virtual representation of the garments has been chosen.

However the look of the body silhouette on the sketches is conducted by the beauty ideal of that time. The post war period is characterized by the typical wasp waist. In virtual space it becomes possible to model the body according to overstated temporal tendencies since the body is merely a hull of Polygons. In the range between a very realistic and a more abstract body, a design towards the aesthetic of the sketches was chosen for the virtual mannequin. The waist is exaggerated unnatural slim, mixed with a typical feminine curved body of the 1940s (Fig. 4.29).

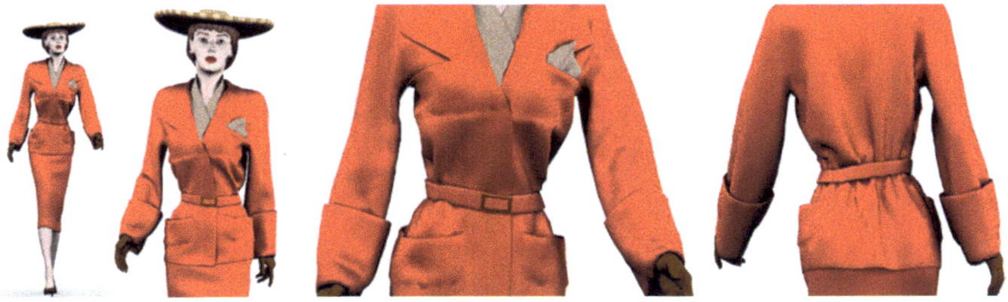

Fig. 4.28 Example orange wool dress

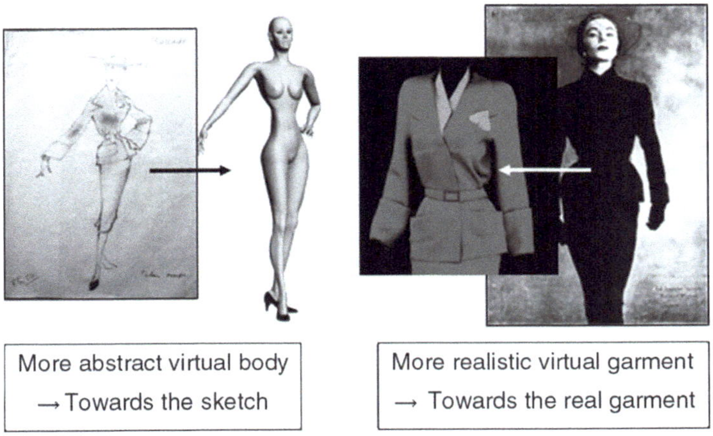

Fig. 4.29 Inspiration for the design of the virtual bodies and dresses

4.8.4.5 Animation

The realistic clothing animation is simulated according to the movement of the virtual actor. This is possible thanks to the collision detection and friction with the surface of the body. The adjustments of simulation parameters can be different from those used during the process of seaming and assembling of the garment. Mechanical simulation gives the realism to the animation of clothing on the virtual mannequin (Fig. 4.30).

For the exhibition Robert Piguet, poses have been recorded according to the sketches, allowing a direct association of the virtual garment with the drawings. In addition, natural walks have been recorded (Fig. 4.31).

4.8.4.6 Final Composition

The final movie was presented in three main parts, referring to the possible intention and utilization of the gowns: daytime, cocktail and evening. The virtual pictures were calculated on a black background.

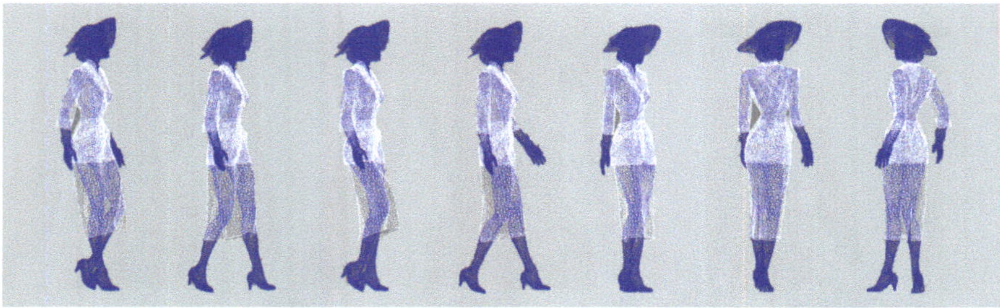

Fig. 4.30 Calculation of the animation

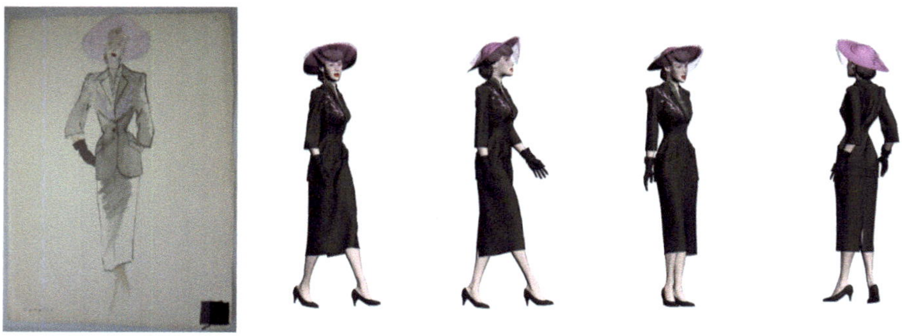

Fig. 4.31 Animation of a sketch of Hubert de Givenchy

4.8.5 Result

Ancient High Fashion garments have been simulated and animated with a highly multifunctional virtual garment design tool and its versatility for complex historic garments has been demonstrated. Based on this experience, new applications for those tools can be thought. Virtual simulations of historic high fashion clothes, which basic constraint is their physical fragility, would preserve them for the next generations, including all their cultural information.

The sketches served the purpose of a direct procurement of the aesthetic dream of the designer. However only through the virtual simulation of the dresses additional aspects could be mediated. Only by the animation of the ideas of Robert Piguet, a relation to the "today" could be added. The dresses defiled in "real time" in front of the eye of the spectator and became revived. The spectator immersed through the virtual defile into the world of fashion and dreams of the past revived (Fig. 4.32).

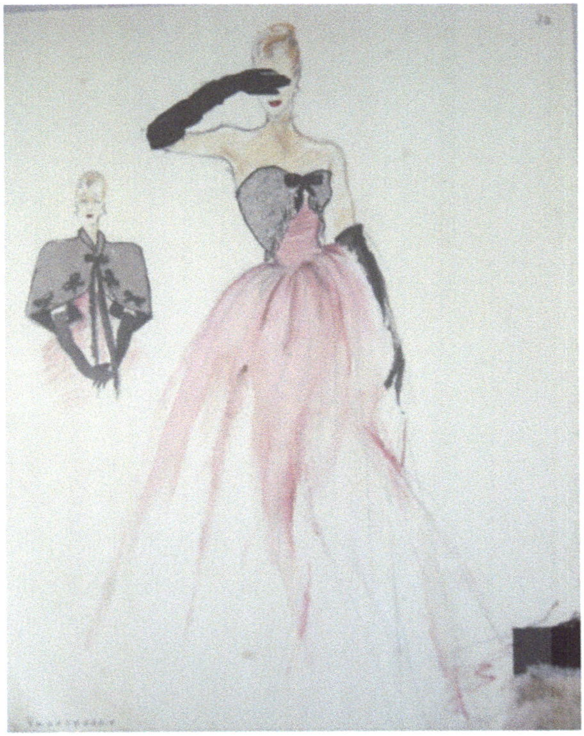

Fig. 4.32 Sketch from Hubert de Givenchy

References

Leardini A., Chiari L., Della Croce U., Cappozzo A.: Human Movement Analysis Using Stereophotogrammetry. Part 3. Soft Tissue Artifact Assessment and Compensation. Gait & Posture, Elsevier, 21:212–225 (2005)

Steele V.: Fifty Years of Fashion: New Look to Now. Yale University Press, ISBN 978-0300087383 (2000)

Volino P., Magnenat-Thalmann N.: Accurate Garment Prototyping and Simulation. Computer-Aided Design and Applications, CAD Solutions, Vol. 2, Issue 5, 645–654 (2005)

Chapter 5
Virtual Prototyping and Collaboration in the Clothing Industry

Abstract This chapter takes a look at the real life application of technologies and techniques as discussed in the previous chapters. The first section discusses the emerging markets and technological trends in the clothing industry with regards to virtual clothing technologies. This is followed by a discussion of virtual garment prototyping. This discussion addresses current design and manufacturing paradigms and the online customization of garments, as well as their associated benefits, limitations and future challenges that need to be tackled. A practical example of such online customization is demonstrated by means of MIRALab's Virtual Try On. The chapter ends with a discussion of the importance of collaboration in the production of garments, addressing such topics as Product Data Management, Product Lifecycle Management and co-design. This is followed by a technical proposal of a virtual garment platform enabling co-design, ranging from low-level communication to higher level user-management.

5.1 Introduction

For many of us technology and broadband connectivity lead to an "on demand" lifestyle where everything everywhere all the time is both expected and desired. The world of clothing and fashion express this "on demand" expectation with advanced garment customization features such as personalized design, fit and fabric performance. This situation has been addressed by a number of R&D projects and industry led innovations and has resulted in new production processes and platforms, the disappearance of intermediaries, higher IT productivity, and new distribution systems. In this context the introduction of virtual clothing technologies propose to innovate and benefit the apparel design and manufacturing landscape in several ways. Agents, product managers, designers, pattern makers and lately consumers (Fig. 5.1) benefit from technologies like garment collection planning, digital editing processes, intuitive user-centric interfaces, 2D pattern annotation, 3D body scanners, 3D garment modeling, simulation and visualization.

N. Magnenat-Thalmann (ed.), *Modeling and Simulating Bodies and Garments*,
DOI 10.1007/978-1-84996-263-6_5,

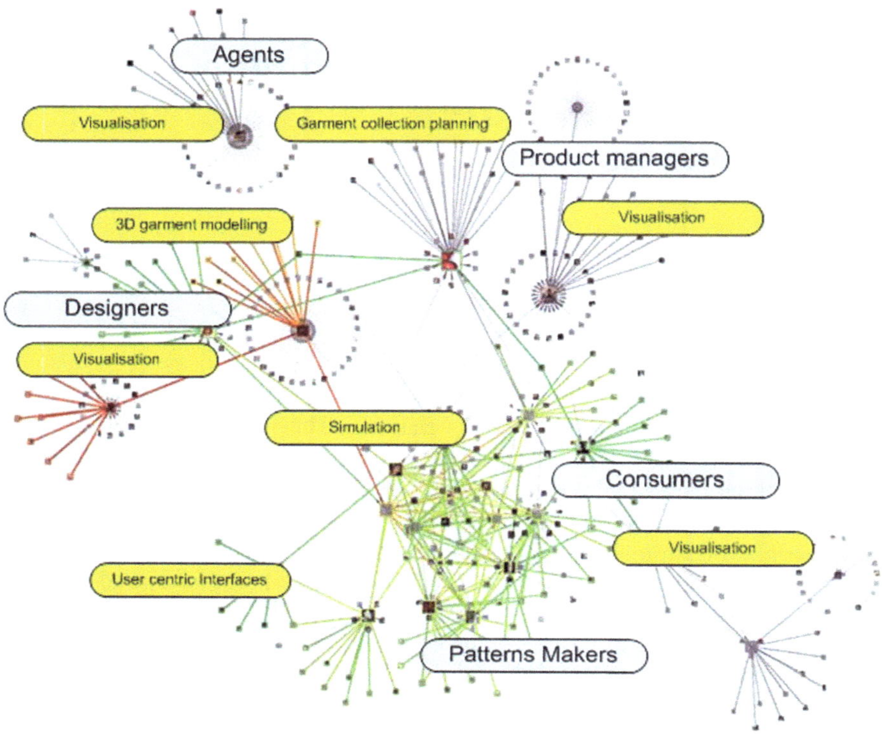

Fig. 5.1 Actors who benefit from virtual clothing technologies

Furthermore companies now recognize that people increase their efforts to interact and socialize online, something that has been pushed significantly by the recent explosion of web2.0 sites and social networks. While the level of online consumer interactivity with the clothing companies increases, this gradually transforms the passive consumer to what is known as a "prosumer" i.e., a producer-consumer, and generates a more "direct economy", where the consumers are drawn, willingly or not, inside the garment production process.

Towards these goals, virtual clothing technologies have provided an added value to the clothing industry on one hand by providing novel production paradigms, such as "Virtual prototyping" and "Virtual Try On", and on the other hand by integrating the user deeper into the design and the operation of the garment manufacturing process through online collaboration platforms. However, today the clothing industry is still taking a limited advantage of the existing virtual clothing technologies to satisfy the current trends to varying degrees. The following examples illustrate clearly the current technological problem the clothing manufacturers need to address today in order to improve their competitive position: for the creation of the virtual prototype of a t-shirt, the simplest form of a 3D garment, a designer needs to spend at least 30 min to 1 h on manual operations, including manual pattern placement and setting the sewing instructions in 2D and/or 3D space. Virtual prototypes of more complex garments, having more pattern pieces, can take up to 1 day to assemble in 3D. Moreover manufacturers take limited advantage of consumer's body shapes, where garment production is based on pre-defined pattern sizes (e.g. XS, S, M, L, XL, XLL) and any bespoke (i.e. advanced personalized) garment manufacturing that is able to serve the masses is still unaccomplished.

In the remaining of this chapter we will elaborate into the emerging marketing and technological trends of the clothing industry with relation to virtual clothing technologies. We will review the concepts of virtual prototyping, virtual try on and online collaboration, their associated benefits and limitations, and the future challenges that need to be tackled. We introduce virtual garment co-design, a concept currently at the research level that brings real-time virtual garment design within networked communities. To this end we describe our approach for the design of the platform architecture.

5.2 The New Market Trend

The last decade the new environment of the "fashion prosumer" has generated demands for tailor-make products for individual customers at a cost comparable to mass production. Hence the mass-customization (MC) and made-to-measure (MtM) segments in the clothing industry have emerged and seek the development of new market opportunities based on product customization combined with the traditional creativity of designers.

The MC and MtM segments of the clothing industry have grown explosively in the past years. A number of innovative market initiatives have addressed this sustainable trend in the recent past, resulting in a small group of visionary actors in the supply chain opening up this market and proving the potentially very large market demand. Towards the implementation of the MC and the MtM market goals, research on virtual clothing has been dealing for several years with different issues around the concepts of virtual prototyping, virtual try on and collaboration. In the next section we will review the concepts and the associated solutions.

5.3 Virtual Prototyping of Garments

Virtual garment simulation is the result of a combination of many techniques that have dramatically evolved during the last decade. The central pillar of garment simulation remains the development of efficient mechanical simulation models, which can accurately reproduce the specific mechanical properties of cloth. However, cloth is by nature highly deformable and specific simulation problems arise from this fact.

In the past, research within the E-Tailor EU project has focused on the mechanical representation of the cloth that should be accurate enough to deal with the nonlinearities and large deformations occurring at any place in the cloth, such as folds and wrinkles. Moreover, the garment cloth interacts strongly with the body that wears it, as well as with the other garments of the apparel. This has required advanced methods for efficiently detecting the geometrical contacts constraining the behavior of the cloth and integrating them into the mechanical model (collision detection and response). All these methods required advanced and complex computational methods where most important key issues remain computation speed and efficiency. Currently the Leapfrog IP EU project is focusing on the real-time simulation issues, where only specific approximation and simplification methods allow the computation of garment animation, trading off some of the mechanical accuracy of the result for visual realism. To this end Leapfrog IP is proposing a real-time garment simulation, animation and resizing (body and cloth) framework.

5.3.1 Current Design and Manufacturing Paradigms

Since 2003, CAD producers started to be very preoccupied by enhancing the way pattern design is made. Three lines of software developing emerged from this:

1. Companies that decided to create some artistic drawing and sketching software (see Fig. 5.2), with the ability to fill the areas with different fabric textures, to add effects and shadows and trying to create by this a realistic view of the final cloth. This approach has obvious limitations: the most important is that there are no connections between the real patterns and the artistic sketch. This line of software is, of course, easy to develop, and it was initially welcomed by the market, but finally proved to be a failure.

   The focus in this case is placed on the designers and the graphic designers who want to create their ready-to-wear collections. Such solutions help also patterns makers and product managers in creating the technical packs for each product of the collection.
2. Companies and Universities that decided to create 2D-to-3D cloth simulation, using a draping/simulation 3D engine that allows user to see how the final product fits on a body (Fig. 5.3) with certain dimensions, and even to produce animated sequences with this product, like a virtual fashion show.

   The large technology providers in the clothing industry (e.g. Lectra, Gerber and Assyst) have developed extensions of their 2D CAD software to include 3D simulation. Even if now the results of these methods are still not satisfying (both technical and in term of market success), the potential is huge, and it is backup by the evolution of computer power. In the area of 2D-to-3D, MIRALab has developed Fashionizer, a system able to provide interactive virtual garment prototyping and fitting. The high level of interactivity required by the features provided in Fashionizer necessitates simultaneous computation of the 3D garment updated immediately to each design modification done to the patterns.

   Fashionizer solution includes a dual view of the garment, featuring both the 2D view of the pattern shapes cut on the fabric and the 3D view of the garment

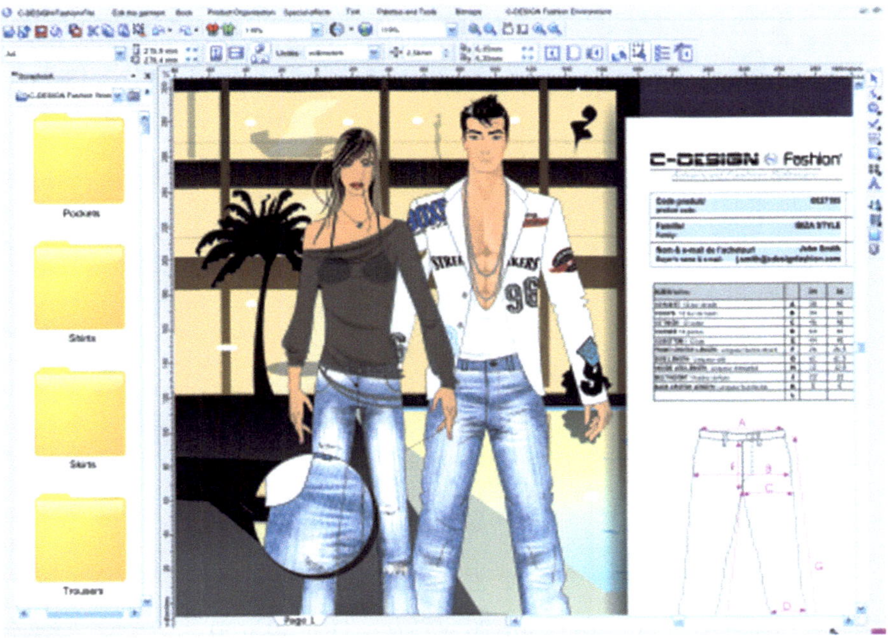

Fig. 5.2 From sketches to technical packages, designers work with drawings/sketches

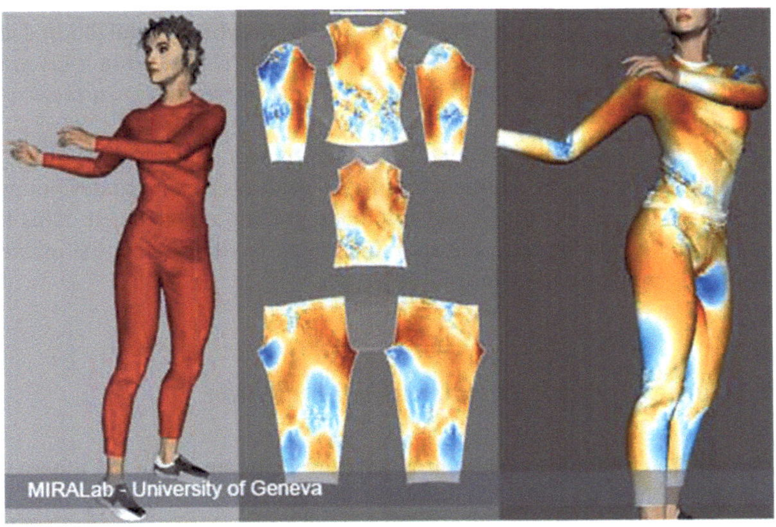

Fig. 5.3 Fashionizer by MIRALab University of Geneva: Fit/Comfort feedback

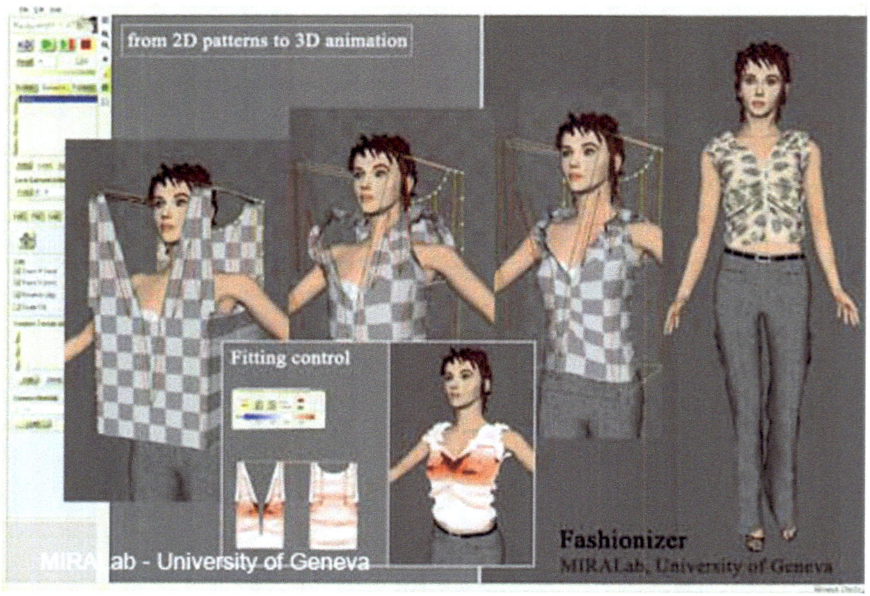

Fig. 5.4 Fashionizer by MIRALab University of Geneva: From 2D to 3D

worn by a virtual character, with tight synchronization (Fig. 5.4). Any editing task carried out in one view is directly displayed in the other view. The system features a fast constrained Delaunay triangulation scheme that allows the discretization of complex patterns described as polygonal lines of control points (2D locations on the fabric). The system allows variable discretization densities over the mesh, as well as size anisotropy (elements elongated in a given direction), for representing adaptively complete garments from large surfaces to intricate details.

3. Companies that remained oriented to 2D environment, and developed their products on this direction, by adding a lot of new methods of pattern developing and altering, new powerful M-t-M and automatic grading methods, etc. This line or development is now more fertile and offers good feedback from the market, but in the long term is clearly limited.

5.3.2 *Current Online Garment Customization*

The Internet along with the rapidly growing power of computing has emerged as a compelling channel for sale of garments. A number of initiatives have arisen recently across the world, revolving around the concepts of Virtual Try On (VTO) and shopping via the Internet. These initiatives are fueled by the current Web tech-

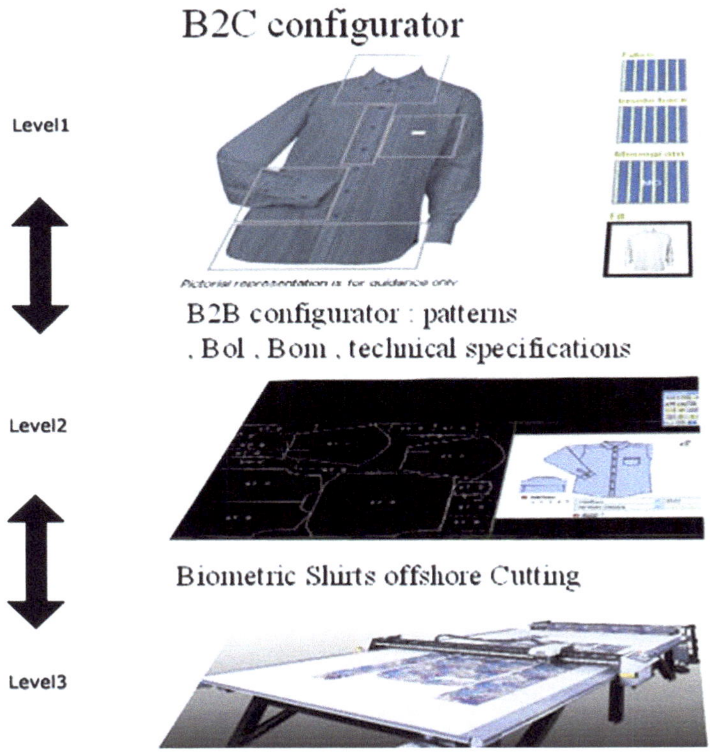

Fig. 5.5 Bivolino 2.5D configurator overview

nologies available, providing an exciting and aesthetically pleasing interface to the general public. However, until now such Web applications have supported only basic functions, such as viewing apparel items in 2,5D combining different items together, mix and match of color and texture, sometimes with a mannequin adjusted to the shopper's proportions.

Existing online M-t-M solutions (Bivolino.com, Fig. 5.5) include 2,5D custom fit configurations (done by the customer) linked with the 2D patterns (on the back office). Other commercial VTO applications focus on static pre-defined garments (e.g. MyVirtualModel, Fig. 5.6) that were previously simulated by the designer.

5.3.3 MIRALab's Virtual Try On

Although current online garment customization and evaluation solutions provide the consumer with helpful tools for their online shopping experience, they cannot replace the physical experience of trying on garments for fit. Solutions such as those mentioned in Section 5.3.2 offer information about style and allow the con-

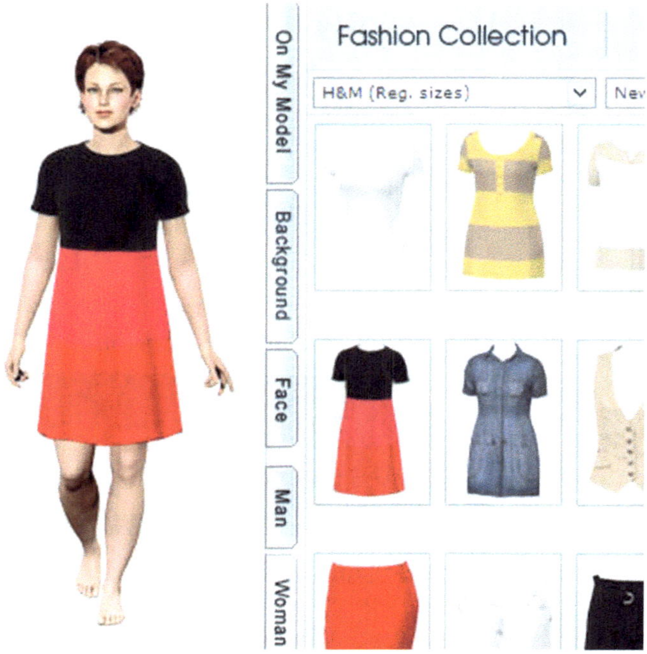

Fig. 5.6 My Virtual Model, online customization

sumer to quickly try out combinations of garments, offering a visual evaluation with regards to style and whether or not certain garments combine well. Any feedback with regards to the fit of a garment, the appropriateness of the selected garment size or the behavior of the selected garment in dynamic everyday scenarios (walking, sitting, or other physical activities) is not provided.

Ideally a good VTO emulates the physical experience of trying on garments as close as possible. Although this physical experience will most likely never be completely replaced by a virtual application, the consumer can still be provided with more information about garment fit and behavior through utilization of a correct mix of the body sizing, motion retargeting and garment simulation technologies as described in the first three chapters. In summary this updated definition of what makes a good VTO leads to three main requirements:

- The used virtual body should have dimensions matching those of the consumer.
- The garments should be physically simulated based on accurately measured physical parameters to allow for the evaluation of dynamic garment behavior as well as garment fit.
- The virtual body should be animatable in order to evaluate garment behavior in dynamic scenarios.

With these requirements in mind we set out to create a VTO that brings us closer to realistic garment evaluation. The main functionality of our VTO is formed by a

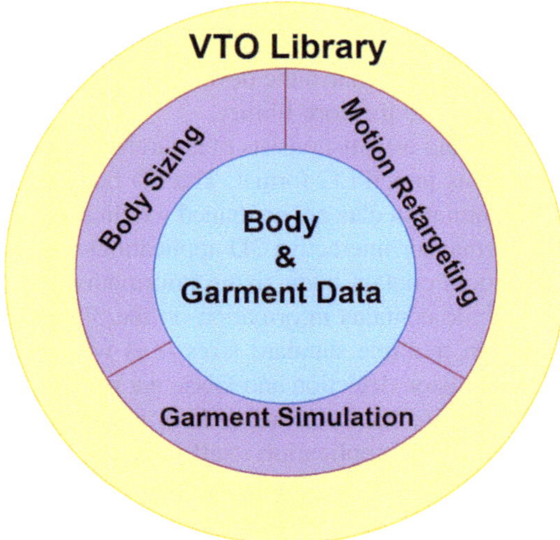

Fig. 5.7 Layered structure of the VTO library

single dynamic library as illustrated in Fig. 5.7, which has been developed in C++. Conceptually data is at the core of the library. This data consists of a textured template body mesh which in combination with the contained motion capture data can be animated. There is furthermore garment data consisting of a 3D garment mesh and some additional information such as fabric parameters and other data.

Around this data-core there are three components that operate on the data. There is a body sizing module which, based on included anthropometric data, can resize the template body to any desired size within a certain range as. A motion retargeting module takes care of the adaptation of the included motion-captured animation to any new morphology specified with the body resizing module. A garment simulation module takes care of the physical simulation of 3D garments based on measured fabric parameters.

The three described libraries in essence work independently from each other on a common set of data and are unaware of the other libraries. It is therefore necessary to introduce a controller that, based on input from the user or based on events such as timer updates, makes the appropriate calls to the individual libraries in the right order. We therefore introduce an outer layer that fulfills exactly this task. It provides a simple interface to the developer with basic interaction functionality (loading new garments, controlling the animation, resizing specific body parts, etc.). The actual details of necessary calls to the different APIs, as well as data organization and exchange are hidden by this layer, significantly simplifying application development.

The main advantage of such a system setup is the ease of deployment of the VTO library in various application scenarios. All the developer has to do is to provide a rendering context and user interface into which the VTO library can be plugged. As a result the same library can be used in a stand-alone application, an ActiveX control for inclusion into a website, as a remote rendering and simulation application or within any other scenario the developer might come up with, without having to make any changes to the core library.

The body and garment data usually consists of a number of files. There are textures for both body and garments in a JPEG format. The 3D body mesh and 3D garment meshes as well as their animation data are contained within a standard Collada, which is an interchange file format for interactive 3D applications. Some minor extensions were made so the file could contain body sizing information, all in a non-standard-breaking manner. A last file contains information on the 3D garments in relation to their pattern – possibly in multiple standard sizes – as well as some precomputed information needed for collision detection and fabric parameters.

In Fig. 5.8 the VTO library has been included in a stand-alone application that can run on the client's PC. The application itself provides and OpenGL rendering context through the use of OpenSceneGraph, an open source high performance 3D graphics toolkit, into which the VTO library is plugged.

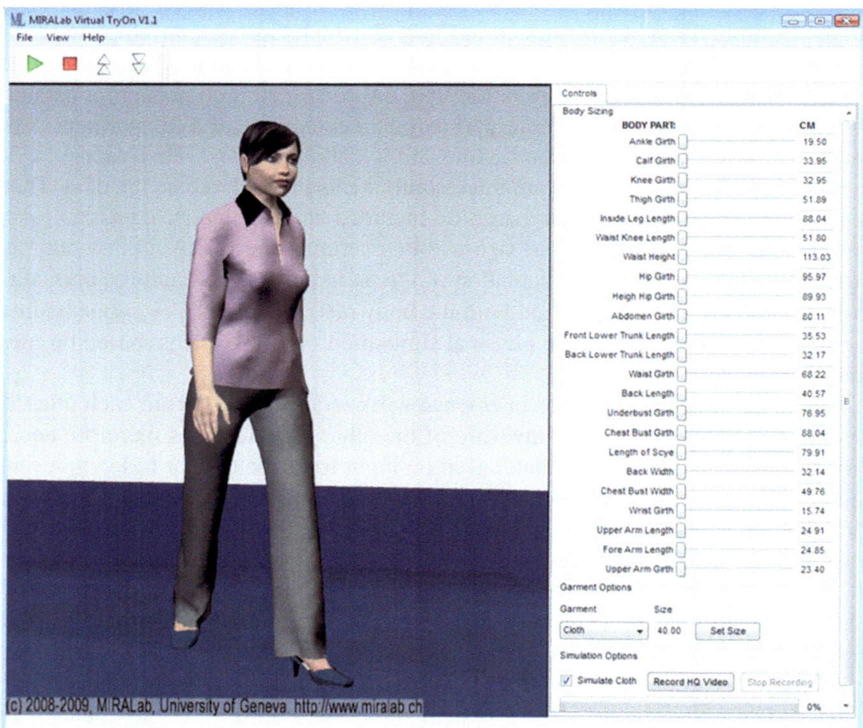

Fig. 5.8 The virtual try on standalone application in action

This application allows the consumer to load a body and garments either by selecting them on their computer or through automatic downloads of a compressed archive containing all files. The body can then be interactively resized, either when the body is at rest, or even during the animation. When the garments have been prepared with patterns at different standard sizes then grading information is also available. This allows the user to dynamically switch between different garment sizes by selecting the size he or she wants to evaluate. The advantage is that no additional information needs to be loaded, nor do we need to switch 3D garment meshes.

In contrast to some available commercial solutions, our VTO contains an interactive and dynamic fully three-dimensional environment. This allows the user to view the model from any desired angle.

In the initial interactive mode the garments are simulated using a quasi-static approach. For more accurate simulation a non-real-time dynamic simulation mode is available. This mode allows the VTO to accurately compute dynamic garment behavior – using the animated virtual model – in mere minutes. Combined with video recording functionality the application delivers a high-quality video to the user of the physically simulated garments. This video can then be viewed at the user's discretion or shared with anyone else.

5.4 Collaboration in Virtual Clothing

Because of ever quicker production cycles, the ability to collaborate and share information is an essential success factor in the fashion industry. Product Data Management (PDM) and Product Lifecycle Management (PLM) solutions are important tools to manage those collaborated processes. PDM/PLM systems enable enterprises to manage and organize data by putting it together in a single environment. Besides stocking all information together, PDM/PLM system also coordinate all product aspects during its lifecycle, from the initial concept to its eventual disposal.

5.4.1 Distinction Between PDM and PLM

The PDM is a component that provides the tools to control access, structure and manage all products' technical data such as geometric models, plans, documentation, texts, drawings or CAD folders. PDM also maintains all information, which is related to a product in a single database (Figs. 5.9 and 5.10).

On the other hand PLM brings together all information related to a product, from the first idea of the product until its disposal. PLM solutions hence accompany the entire products lifecycle and allow a later share and access of data. A product's lifecycle is divided into four stages: introduction, growth, maturity and decline.

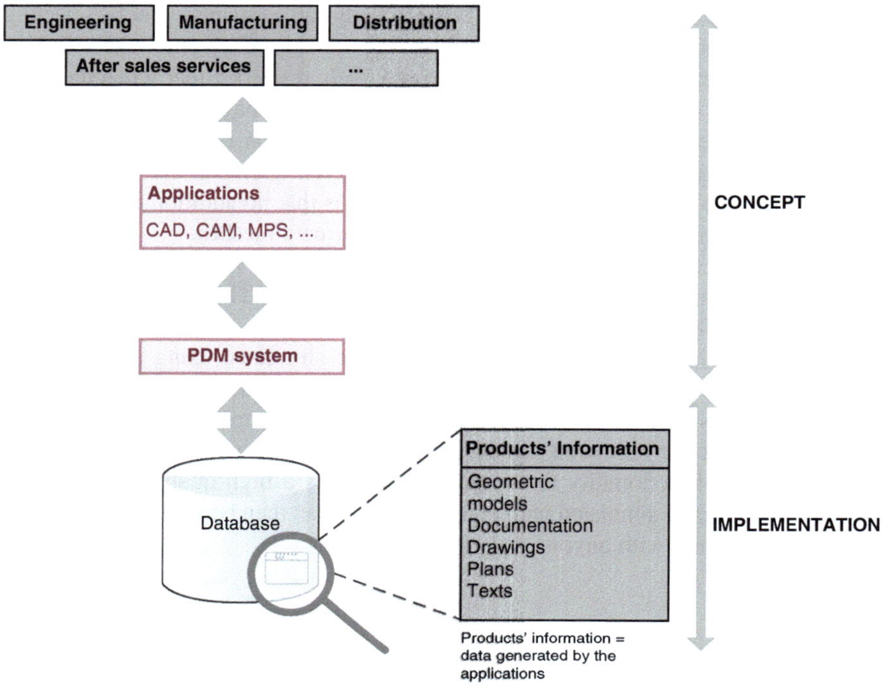

Fig. 5.9 Scheme of the PDM solution

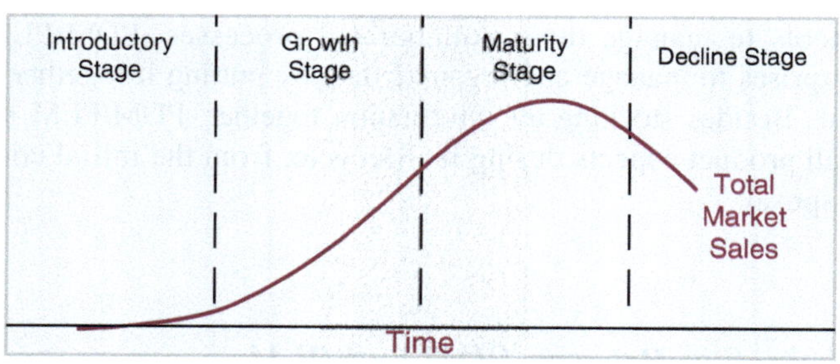

Fig. 5.10 Evaluation of the product sales upon four different stages

In the introductory stage, enterprises build the product and develop a market for it. In the growth stage, enterprises try to increase product market share. In the maturity stage, enterprises have to protect the product market share in order to avoid competition and maximize profit and in the final stage, the sales decline. At each stage, enterprises have various options: they can maintain the product, discontinue it or improve it.

5.4.2 *PDM/PLM in the Apparel Industry: Current Solutions/ Examples and Their Benefits*

In the apparel industry, the main aim of PDM/PLM solutions is to maintain and improve the garment collection management and product development processes. PDM/PLM applications bring together all numeric data, related to a garment product and its processes, in one single environment and hence, all information will be stocked in one database. Like this, PDM/PLM systems allow a better response to customers' requirements, an enhanced planning of processes and a reduction of cost and time. In the end, products time to market are improved, one of the most critical aspects of garment development processes and companies using PDM/PLM solutions stay in competition.

Lectra, one of the leading CAD/CAM companies, offers a web-based PDM/PLM solution. With the use of PDM/PLM solutions, companies such as Mango were finally able to better coordinate their multiple product lines, implying the management of an increasing number of personnel and duties. In the future, Lectra aims to link their PDM/PLM solutions with other Lectra design and modeling applications in order to optimize again the collection development processes. Important features will be a better link to trend tables and to virtual 3D visualization applications.

Gerber is another leading CAD/CAM company offering the solution WebPDM and FLM (Fashion Lifecycle Management). Both solutions are again Web-based and hence, easy to use. Their main focus is the reduction of time consuming product development cycles and the improvement of communication problems. The CAD/ CAM Company Assyst-Bullmer provides PDM/PLM solutions since 10 years. More recently they introduced new, more flexible solutions, pdm.assyst and plm. complete. Other PDM/PLM solutions, specialized for the apparel industry, are provided by Circon, Geac RunTime, MatrixOne, World fashion exchange (WFX).

In general all solutions have the same goal: To solve and improve the companies strategic and operational needs. Solutions promise to handle increasing market demands, to reduce the product development time and cost and to better manage the product development data. However, the different solutions also have some fine distinctions regarding their objectives and thus attract different customers. Lectra is counting 17,000 customers today, located in more than 100 countries. Assyst-Bullmer currently has around 7,000 customers worldwide and MatrixOne was chosen by approximately 850 customers, among them GAP.

5.5 Future Challenge: Co-design

The term co-design is used in the literature with regards to cooperation between a firm and its individual customers during the configuration process of a customised product. Customer co-design describes a process that allows customers to express their product requirements and carry out product realization processes by mapping the requirements into the physical domain of the product. The co-design option, although quite an intriguing concept in principle, it has not still reached its full potential and in many cases can create confusion to consumers if they are left alone to decide what configuration suits best their preferences, somatotypes and lifestyle. It has been shown that consumers often are attracted by the additional value of a custom product. This value, however, often is counterbalanced by the perceived complexity of fulfilling the configuration task. Towards this end, the desire of customers to use co-design services not only to create a unique design, but also as an exciting experience (e.g. by virtually trying-on the items designed by them, or asking the advise of a stylist or a friend) should be taken seriously into account.

Mass-customizers should seriously consider experience aspects and environmental stimulation when developing a mass customization project, especially if they are operating online. Addressed to the end-consumer, but also used as source of valuable information for New Configurable Product Development and CRM (Customer Relationship Management). CCD will be accompanied by an on-line community, an innovative 3D Product Configurator, and VTO (Virtual Try-On). This will enable the visualization of selected configurations of customizable items on a virtual mannequin that resembles the body conformation of the customer, with comfort and fit information overlayed.

Towards this goal, the new EU project SERVIVE aims to develop knowledge-based web services that will relate to style expertise, human body expertise and data, material and specific manufacturing knowledge. The Servive will also enable all necessary interactions of customers with value-chain actors, thus enabling and encouraging the active participation of end consumers in the configuration of the customized items. The selected product configuration will in turn influence the production scenario. In the following sections we are going to describe MIRALab's approach for the design and implementation of a real time collaboration platform for co-design purposes.

5.6 Towards a Co-design Virtual Garments Platform

As the Internet has become a common infrastructure to connect lots of users interacting with each other with various way of sharing their contexts, it is becoming prevalent to develop multi-user applications in both academic and industrial societies such as instant messaging services, multi-user online games, networked virtual communities and so on. Among such promising applications is the co-design virtual garments system. This major trend also makes existing stand-alone applications for single user be extended and evolved to ones for multiple users. If an application developer wants to develop a multi-user system or change a single-user application for the multiple-user purpose, he/she has to take into consideration not only intrinsic functionalities of the system but also how each system can be connected and communicate with each other to support multiple users. To realize this, he/she could do pure socket level network programming or use other application level communication toolkit or middleware. However, in the case of socket level programming, application developers have to take care of everything relating to communication from the low level socket management to the high level aspect of distributed user interaction. Although there have been existing communication middleware systems which provide high level wrappers of basic functionalities for network programming, they still need to be improved in terms of easy and simple development of multi-user systems. In one hand, some communication environments still put many responsibilities to developers instead of supporting diversities of fundamental communication means. On the other hand, other toolkits are focus on specific applications and it is difficult to use them for another systems. For supporting developers, it is a dilemma how to balance between the freedom and simple way of the development.

In this section, we discuss a common collaborative platform which enables developers to make multi-user applications in an easy and simple way considering a common step to implement them. Especially, we focus on the interaction technologies based on underlying networked collaboration. Therefore, the proposed platform is designed not only for the co-design virtual garments system described in previous sections but also any kind of multi-user applications. To realize this purpose, we extract general requirements to develop an application for multiple users in terms of communication architecture, user membership management, event management, message delivery and process and support for transmission of various contents. The proposed collaborative platform which is separated from application provides high level APIs to support required functionalities. It consists of three main manager modules: communication manager, event manager and node manager. The communication manager manages communication channels created by applications and provides send/receive methods of different socket wrappers of TCP and UDP, file, and multimedia communication. The event manager converts application level events created by application to low level messages that are transmitted by the communication manager. When a message is delivered from the communication manager to the event manager, it parses the message to an application event and forwards it to both the node manager and application so that they can handle the event. The node manager handles received events internally and automatically manages user membership in different hierarchy. All the three managers are integrated with an intermediate stub module which directly interacts with an application layer. Developers use the stub module for high level control of the platform or also can access each manager module for low level functionalities if needed.

An overall structure of a communication node integrated with the collaborative platform is easily set by a configuration file in which we can set the communication role of the application (server or client), session management (multiple sessions or single session) and user membership control (no user authentication or authentication by application).

5.6.1 Related Work

In this section, we discuss and analyze several middleware tools which help users develop distributed and multi-user applications by providing various functionalities with different goals and views.

Adaptive Communication Environment (ACE) (Schmidt and Huston 2003) is an open-source object-oriented framework that implements many core patterns for concurrent communication software. ACE is designed to help developers of high-performance and real-time communication applications. It provides a rich set of software modules such as event de-multiplexing and event handler dispatching, signal handling, service initialization, inter-process communication, shared memory management, message routing, dynamic configuration of distributed services, and concurrent execution and synchronization. ACE simplifies a way of developing network applications. However, it still puts much responsibility on developers to develop a multi-user purpose application because they focus more on software modules which concern an efficient way of managing relatively low level signal, process, thread and socket. Using ACE, developers still have to take care of and implement how communication architecture and user membership management should be in their network application.

Common Object Request Broker Architecture (CORBA) (Object Management Group 2001) is an architecture standardized by Object Management Group (OMG) which enables software components in a same application or a remote host in a network to interact with each other. Developers use an interface definition language (IDL) to specify the interfaces through which objects communicate by a way of normal method call. It also supports multiple languages such as C, C++, Java, Python, etc. Interfaces de-fined by developers are required to be converted into language-specific classes to interfacing with CORBA infrastructure. While CORBA provides a standardized and normalized means of easy way for objects in distributed systems to communicate, developers who would like to make a distributed application should have additional knowledge of the internal CORBA architecture, components and proto-cols. Because of problems incurred by the heavy and complex specifications of CORBA, developers devised Internet Communications Engine (ICE) (Henning 2004) which has similar functionalities but is much lighter than CORBA. It, however, supports various ways of RPC style object interaction which is relatively low level supports and still overlooks much higher level of requirements for multi-user systems.

SOAP (SOAP 2004) is a message passing protocol for exchanging XML-based messages using HTTP/HTTPS and is widely used in Web applications which provide Web services. SOAP also uses RPC style messaging pattern in which client sends a request message to another communication node (server or client) and the recipient node handles the request and immediately sends a response to the client. As SOAP uses application layer transport protocols such as HTTP and SMTP, it allows relatively easier way of transmitting messages rather than transport layer protocols (e.g. TCP and UDP). But there have been critics about the performance due to verbose XML message format. In our view, it also does not provide any high level features required for efficient support of distributed multi-user applications because it is originally designed as a messaging protocol, not a middleware or toolkit level.

While aforementioned middleware and protocols provide developers with a way of communicating nodes in a relatively low level manner, there are also many application level middleware approaches which supports different application specific functionalities according to specific needs for multi-user systems. Among compelling multi-user applications are online games and many research works (Morgan et al. 2005; Broll et al. 2006; Balan et al. 2005) have devised dedicated middleware and technical schemes that are tightly coupled with their own games. We also have many open source or proprietary game engines supporting multi-user capability (e.g. OLIVE, Ca3DE; DimensioneX; CrystalSpace; Ogre3D), but most of them focus on 3D graphics engine and various components stuck to game application and provide still limited networking support with fixed client/server model. Even though such middleware approaches support well customized functionalities meeting their own requirements, it is not suitable to use them in other multi-user applications that have different purposes.

5.6.2 Design Considerations

When we design a middleware or architecture with a layered approach, there is a trade-off between the freedom of users and simplicity of development as discussed in the previous section. In one hand, when we provide only low-level functions and put most responsibilities to users, they have more freedom to develop and improve functionalities using the provided functions. However instead, they should take care of all details of the new implemented modules. On the other hand, if a system provides users with simple APIs which have such high-level functionalities, it makes developers implement a module in an efficient way. In this case, however, they are sometimes restricted to have more flexibility to change the sup-ported modules which have limited number of possible options. Extremely speaking, this is the problem of using a pure programming language or a high-level toolkit. Therefore, in this section, we focus on multi-user applications possibly in general and analyze fundamental requirements which could efficiently benefit developers both with high and low level features.

From the experience of work on network framework for distributed virtual environments (DVEs) (Lee et al. 2007), we have found several fundamental features required for developing multi-user systems as following sub-sections.

5.6.3 Communication Architecture

Depending on how the communication between users (or end nodes) is coordinated, its architecture can be characterized as illustrated in Fig. 5.11: client/server, peer/peer and peer/server.

In the client/server architecture, communication between users has to be done via a server. To interact with other users, each user should transmit his messages to the server which then forwards them to other users. This architecture benefits a simple consistency and security mechanism for which the server is responsible.

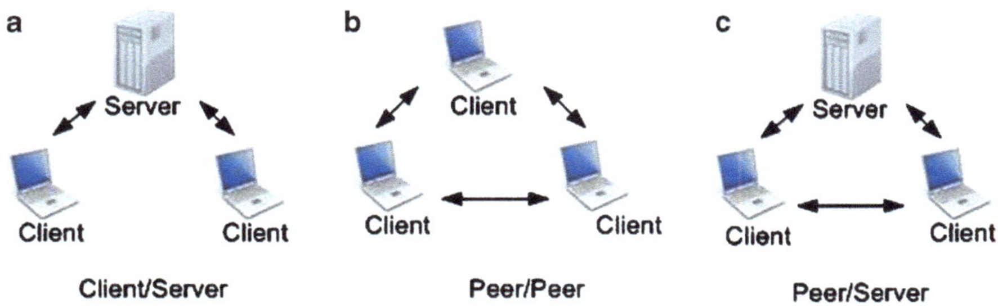

Fig. 5.11 Communication architecture

The server can perform efficient message filtering by forwarding data to only selected receivers according to their interests, for instance. However, this architecture has scalability problems. First, since all the messages among users must pass through the server, they require one additional hop to reach the receivers, which can increase delay in transmission time. Second, when the server fails to operate, all clients connected to the server cannot interact with each other until the server recovers. Finally, as the number of clients connected to the server increases, it may become a performance bottleneck. In spite of the problems described above, successful massively multiplayer online games (MMOGs) (e.g. Lineage2; World of Warcraft) adopt the client/server architecture as their communication architecture, since it can efficiently keep the system consistent and be well deployed in the current Internet without multicast capability. For scalability, some systems introduce multiple servers to overcome the limit in one server in terms of the number of clients and a single point of failure.

In the peer/peer architecture, there is no server involved in the communication between clients. Thus, no single point of failure problem exists. Even if some clients fail to operate, the rest can interact transparently. The clients can interact with each other via a direct communication channel. Since there exists no server maintaining a consistent state, each client host is responsible for keeping its state consistent with others. This imposes a burden on the client. Especially if unicast communication is used, each client has to maintain as many connections as the number of other clients with which it intends to interact. The more clients exist, the more connections are required. That is, the scalability problem occurs. Multicast communication is used to avoid this problem in the peer/peer architecture where each user maintains only one multicast address assigned to the group which he or she is interested in. While multicast can reduce the communication overhead, fine-grained message filtering such as filtering per user is not possible as in the unicast communication. Another problem of multicast is its slow deployment in the Internet due to various reasons. In addition to linking multicast islands via Mbone (Macedonia and Brutzman 1994) and adding more control functionalities to the tunnel end points, application level multicast (Hosseini and Georganas 2004) has been proposed as an alternative solution without native IP multicast. Early adoption of IPv6 may make multi-cast become a reality in the Internet.

The Peer/peer architecture is used by file sharing applications (e.g. Gnutella, Kazaa) although some of them are not pure Peer/peer but adopts a directory server to improve the performance of file search and management.

The peer/server architecture is a hybrid of the two architectures above. There exists a server like the client/server architecture. The server has a role of managing user membership and maintaining a consistent state of the virtual world. However, users directly communicate with each other using a multicast communication channel like the peer/peer architecture. The server does not redistribute messages, but just receives them and updates the current state by joining corresponding multicast groups. This allows a new comer to get the up-to-dated information of a virtual world from the server instead of multicasting the request for the information when he joins the world. This means that the peer/server architecture adopts the benefits of both the client/server model and the peer/peer model. Because of the deployment problem of multicast, this architecture has been studied mostly by academic researchers.

5.6.4 User Membership Management

As multi-user applications deal with more than one user, membership management is one of crucial feature to be supported in such systems. The membership management enables a system to manage users so that only authorized users can access a system and can know who is registered in a server and who is currently online for any interaction. There are various ways of management depending on total number of users and characteristics of systems. The simplest management is to keep the list of all user information in one repository of the system where users know the whole list of others when they connect to the system (see Fig. 5.12a). As it does not need additional care of user membership management, it can be adopted to applications which have a few users in total such as collaborative design systems (Xu and Liu 2003), video conferencing tools, messenger tools, and other group-ware applications (Masoodian et al. 2005). When a system tries to support lots of users (hundreds or hundred thousands), however, it requires that a system organizes several groups of users for efficient membership management. Users can be grouped in different ways according to the requirement of applications which need to manage lots of users. Some typical multi-user online games support sessions where users join and play with others in the same session. It is the case if a game supports a few numbers of users in one session and enables users to manage their own sessions. When there are a lot of connected users in a server, each of them can create, delete, join and leave sessions, and wait or invite others before starting the game of this session. We regard users in a session as one user group. In this case, a server manages users with groups (sessions) and each group is independent of another, which means that a user can interact only with others in his/her session and a group has no relationship with other groups (see Fig. 5.12b).

In MMOGs, however, lots of (thousands of) users register, connect to a server and play altogether in one virtual environment. Users are grouped in a server level

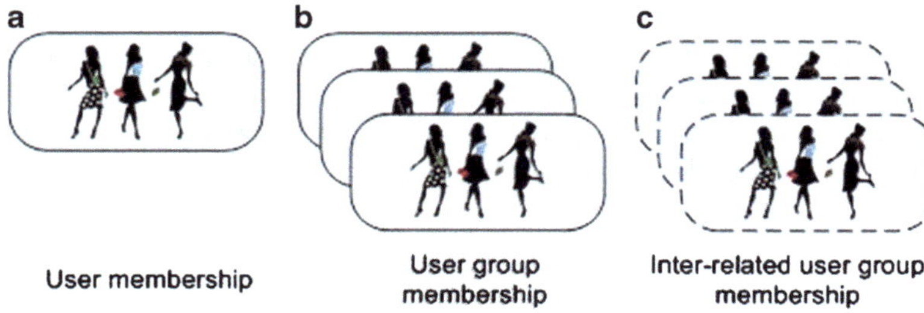

Fig. 5.12 Different membership management

in-stead of session level as they have an option to select in which server they would like to play. Each server operates its own independent world and users in different servers do not interact with each other as the database is separated. In a game world, users can manage a specific type of small group on demand, for example when they want to do a quest with other players. This instant group is similar to session level group management mentioned above. The difference is that it is possible for a group to interact with another group in a way of collaboration or fighting with each other. Figure 5.12c represents this type of user groups.

There are also different concepts of grouping users in multi-user applications such as regions and auras in distributed virtual environments (DVEs), user categories in messenger and social network applications, and so on, and different type of groups can be arranged in different layer as discussed in the case of MMOGs. No matter which name is used for grouping users, the user group is classified into one of above three kinds of groups: one group, independent group and inter-related group.

5.6.5 *Content Transmission Scheme*

When application developers determine the communication architecture and the type of user membership management, we have communicating nodes and multiple users connected with each other somehow. The next step to think to develop a multi-user application is how a node sends and receives a message to its counterpart, which is one of fundamental requirements to make a system work and enable users to interact with each other. A system can provide different types of sending scheme depending on the communication architecture, application needs, number of users, and situation of current network infrastructure. As multiple users have to send and receive messages among them, we put most concern in transmission of a message to more than one user. As discussed in the communication architecture section, sending to multiple users is a common situation in any type of communication architecture. Although the multicast is an efficient way in terms of bandwidth consumption, as it is not commonly used yet because of the problem of deployment and cost model for commercialization, a system should provide an alternative such as multiple unicast transmissions. In addition, combining with the user membership management, more detailed transmissions can be supported. If a system has and manages user groups, the transmission scheme can be limited to such specific groups. For the user group, developers could specify the transmission to a group no matter which transmission scheme is used. The destination of a message could be an individual user, a specific group, a group of groups, or all users. Developers also benefit from this specific transmission scheme when they want to implement a filtering scheme which implies sending/receiving messages only to/from interested users and reducing useless bandwidth consumption of sending to irrelevant users.

Another aspect to be taken into account when we design a multi-user application is which kinds of content are transmitted. A node may send a specific form of content such as an image file, AV stream, 3D data, and so on according to the aim of an application. A collaborative platform could be a more flexible and efficient tool if it provides developers with options of all issues discussed: different transmission schemes and sending/receiving different type of content.

5.6.6 Event Management

In the previous section, we discussed different sending schemes of various kinds of contents. However, it is not enough to make the whole system work. To enable communicating nodes to understand and interact with each other, we need a set of control messages. Otherwise, even though we send/receive a lot of content to/from distant nodes, there is no way to understand what they mean in an application level. Therefore, a multi-user system has to support how to define an *event*[1] which includes a common information (e.g. message size, destination address, message ID, etc.) and application-specific information which it would like to deliver such as user and content information. Every middleware system has its own way of defining an event and fields inside. In most cases, connected nodes communicate via the exchange of the combination of events and content using a request/reply model as illustrated in Fig. 5.13 for an example. If we develop a general collaborative platform, it surely must have means to manage arbitrary events in an efficient way: creation of a new event and deletion of an existing event, for instance. In addition, it requires a structured way from the event definition, creation of a new event and translation to an appropriate form of message for transmission/reception, which is a normal process to handle a communicated event.

5.6.7 Proposed Architecture

In this section, we propose a collaborative platform, CM which takes into consideration on design issues in the previous section. Our approach includes various

[1] An *event* is a high-level form which includes semantics that an application knows, and we use the term, a *message* for a low-level form which is interfaced with underlying network APIs.

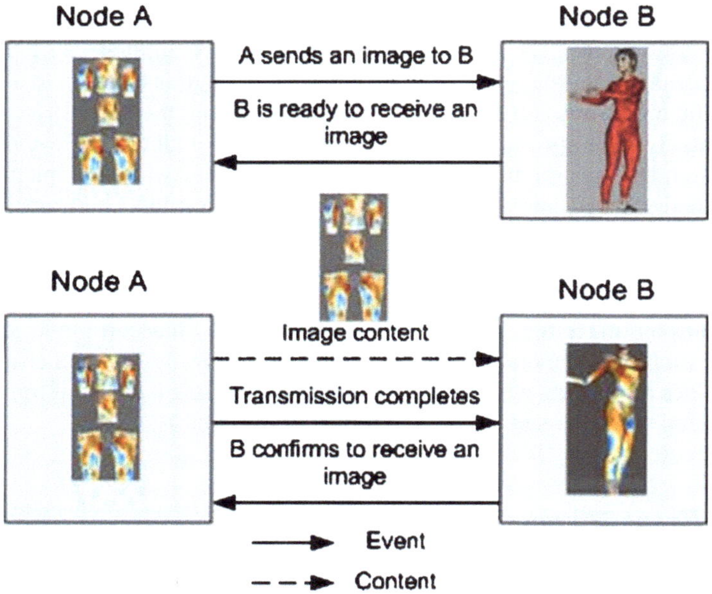

Fig. 5.13 Content and event exchange

features such as communication architecture, user membership management, content transmission and event management, all of which are required for developing multi-user applications.

5.6.8 Overall Architecture

The proposed collaborative platform aims to provide an easy and efficient way of developing a multi-user application. It supports various functionalities with options for different requirements of developers. The platform deals with multi-user issues which have to be implemented by developers if it has only fundamental networking supports. Our system has a role of bridge between an application and underlying network infrastructure. Among basics to do this is to deliver messages and contents between these two entities, by which communicating nodes can interact with each another. With APIs provided by the proposed platform, application developers can create, send, receive, and process an event. In addition to dealing with events, it supports other operations which detect a specialized event and conduct a dedicated service according to the event type. To support them, we follow the layered approach to design the platform. Figure 5.14 shows an overall architecture of the proposed platform. In the point of view of applications, the proposed platform consists of four main modules in order: application stub, node manager, event manager, and communication manager. We describe details of each module in the following sub-sections.

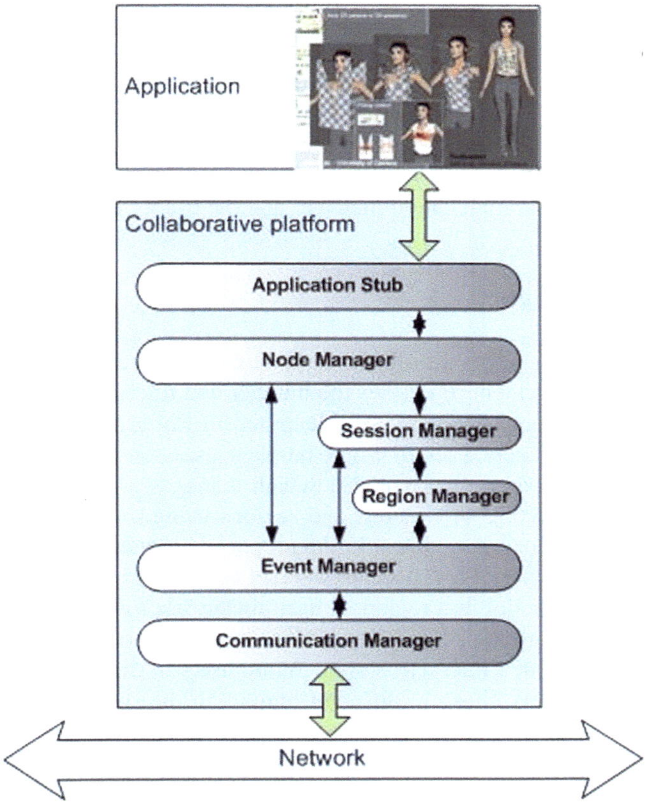

Fig. 5.14 Collaborative platform architecture

5.6.8.1 Application Stub

The application stub is a core module which interfaces an application. A developer can access most of supporting functionalities of the proposed platform with this module. In general, it provides APIs to start and stop the collaborative platform, register and deregister an event to be used among communicating nodes, send an event, and assign an event handling callback function which is called by the system whenever it receives an event from a remote node. All events created in an application and needed to be sent pass through the application stub until the underlying network layer. The application stub then notifies an application of every received event from a remote node through the registered callback function so that the application can deal with incoming events.

In addition to these fundamental operations, depending on the application type (a client or a server) and the communication architecture (client/server, peer-to-peer, or hybrid), which are assigned in a configuration file by a developer, the application stub provides appropriate useful functions with various options. For example, if the application is a client type in the client/server architecture, the application stub offers a function to connect to a server. What a developer has to do is to set the server information like the IP address and port in the configuration file and call the simple connection function. All the rest operations required for creating a new channel, initializing it, and binding addresses are performed by other underlying responsible module such as the communication manager and the event manager.

5.6.8.2 Node Manager

The node manager manages a different level of user interaction area according to the application requirement. It defines the number and relationship of sessions and regions in a hierarchical structure. As illustrated in Fig. 5.14, the node manager contains session managers, each of which handles a session and a session manager can have more than one region manager which manages a region. The developer can organize the structure of sessions and regions using the configuration file or APIs provided by manager modules. In the proposed architecture, we need at least one session and region to allow users to interact with each other. It means that the minimal unit of interaction is a region. A user always has to belong to a region. By default, we define a session as an independent interaction area and regions inside a session as an interrelated interaction area. While users in different session usually do not exchange events, those in different regions in the same session frequently interact with each other. However, this assignment between a session and a region is just logical concept, and a developer can define his/her own relationship among them through APIs. For example, the node manager provides APIs which can distribute an event to different sessions and regions. A developer can assign and distribute an event to specific sessions or regions. In addition, although static configuration of the session and region is given by the configuration file, the manager module also provides functions to manage them dynamically such as creation/deletion of a session or a region. The session and region structure is tightly coupled with the user membership management which we discuss in another section.

An event passing through the application stub module from the application layer stops by the node manager which then checks the destination users in sessions or regions, and delivered to the event manager before being sent. All inbound events from the network are also delivered to the node manager. It checks the event header and does internal process if it is required. If an event handler is a session manager or a region manager, the node manager delivers it to an appropriate manager.

5.6.8.3 Event Manager

The event manager is in charge of an event in the system. An event is a high-level form of exchange method between application nodes. As it includes semantics to be exchanged so that it can be understandable at the application layer, high-level manager modules (the node manager, session manager, and region manager) and an application uses an event as a way of information exchange. One of key role of the event manager is to change an event to a low-level message (sequence of byte array) which is delivered to the underlying communication manager, and vice versa. The event manager provides several event send functions which take an event as a parameter and transform it into a message so that it can be sent via the communication manager. To the contrary, an incoming message given by the communication manager is converted to an event in the event manager which then delivers it to the node manager for the internal operation. The event manager also forwards the converted event to the application stub module which eventually delivers it to an application for the event process at the application layer as well.

5.6.8.4 Communication Manager

The communication manager controls messages and provides APIs to manage communication channels. The main role is to send and receive messages to/from underlying network. To support this, the communication manager runs a separate thread for waiting any incoming message. Whenever it receives a message from the network, the communication manager forwards it to the event manager. It also uses its own send functions embedded in each channel when a message to be sent is delivered from the event manager. If an application creates a channel, it is maintained in the communication manager as a channel list. Every event channel in the list is checked by the receiving thread and any received message is notified to the event manager. Therefore, the communication manager supports asynchronous communication among nodes as it does not guarantee for a channel in the list to receive an immediate reply in a blocking state. However, the collaborative platform also allows a developer to make synchronous communication by managing each channel in a separate way. The system provides different dedicated communication sockets which wrap native socket APIs and makes it possible an easy way to open and close a channel depending on demand. Supported socket types are a server socket, a stream socket, datagram socket, and a multicast socket. The server socket is used in the server side which waits and opens connection with requesting clients. The counterpart of the server socket is the stream socket which is the wrapper of a normal TCP socket. The datagram socket is for UDP connection of either a server or a client. The multicast socket is on top of the datagram socket for multicast communication. It is useful when routers enable multicast routing. Developers can enable the synchronous communication by directly using the wrapper sockets instead of the communication manager.

References

Balan R, Misra A, Ebling M, Castro P: Matrix: Adaptive middleware for distributed multiplayer games. Technical Report RC23764, IBM Research Watson, Hawthorne, NY, (2005)

Broll W, Ohlenburg J, Lindt I, Herbst I, Braun A: Meeting technology challenges of pervasive augmented reality games. In: Proceedings of 5th ACM SIGCOMM workshop on Network and system support for games, Singapore, (2006)
Ca3DE. http://www.ca3d-engine.de/c_Features.php
Collada. http://www.collada.org
Crystal Space. http://www.crystalspace3d.org/main/Main_Page
DimensioneX. http://www.dimensionex.net/en/
Henning M: A new approach to object-oriented middleware. IEEE Internet Computing, Vol. 8, Issue 1, (2004)
Hosseini M, Georganas N. D: End System Multicast Protocol for Collaborative Virtual Environments. Presence: Teleoperators and Virtual Environments, Vol. 13, Issue 3, 263–278, MIT Press (2004)
Lee D, Lim M, Han S, Lee K: ATLAS: A scalable network framework for distributed virtual environments. Presence: Teleoperators and Virtual Environments, Vol. 16, Issue 2, 125–156, (2007)
Lineage2. http://www.lineage2.com/
Macedonia, M. R., Brutzman, D. P: MBone Provides Audio and Video Across the Internet. Computer Vol. 27, Issue 4, 30–36, IEEE Computer Society Press (1994)
Masoodian M, Luz S, Bouamrane M, King D: RECOLED: A group-aware collaborative text editor for capturing document history. In: Proceedings of WWW/Internet 2005, Vol. 1, Lisbon, Portugal, pp. 323–330, (2005)
Morgan G, Lu F, Storey K: Interest management middleware for networked games. In: Proceedings of symposium on Interactive 3D graphics and games, Washington, USA, pp. 57–64, (2005)
Ogre3D. http://www.ogre3d.org/
OpenSceneGraph. http://www.openscenegraph.org
Object Management Group: The Common Object Request Broker: Architecture and Specification (2.4 edition). OMG Technical Committee Document (formal/2001-02-33), (2001)
Schmidt D, Huston S: C++ Network Programming: Systematic Reuse with ACE and Frameworks. Addison-Wesley Longman, (2003)
SOAP Version 1.2 Part 1: Messaging Framework. http://www.w3.org/TR/soap12-part1, (2004)
World of Warcraft. http://www.worldofwarcraft.com/
Xu W, Liu T: A web-enabled PDM system in a collaborative design environment. Robotics and Computer-Integrated Manufacturing, Vol. 19, Issue 4, 315–328(14), Elsevier (2003)

MIX
Papier aus verantwortungsvollen Quellen
Paper from responsible sources
FSC® C105338

If you have any concerns about our products,
you can contact us on
ProductSafety@springernature.com

In case Publisher is established outside the EU,
the EU authorized representative is:
Springer Nature Customer Service Center GmbH
Europaplatz 3, 69115 Heidelberg, Germany

Printed by Libri Plureos GmbH
in Hamburg, Germany